THE
HERSHBERG
DIET

THE
HERSHBERG
DIET

DISCOVER HOW THE 4TH MACRO CAN HELP YOU SHED POUNDS AND BEAT THE METABOLIC SYNDROME

Melissa Hershberg, M.D.

KEY PORTER BOOKS

Library and Archives Canada Cataloguing in Publication

Hershberg, Melissa
   The hershberg diet / Melissa Hershberg.

ISBN-13: 978-1-55263-799-9, ISBN-10: 1-55263-799-9

   1. Reducing diets. 2. Nutrition. 3. Diet. I. Title.

RM222.2.H46 2007   613.2'5   C2006-901816-2

The publisher gratefully acknowledges the support of the Canada Council for the Arts and the Ontario Arts Council for its publishing program. We acknowledge the support of the Government of Ontario through the Ontario Media Development Corporation's Ontario Book Initiative.

We acknowledge the financial support of the Government of Canada through the Book Publishing Industry Development Program (BPIDP) for our publishing activities.

This publication contains the ideas and opinions of the author. The information presented is designed to help you make informed decisions about your health. It is not intended as a substitute for medical advice. Please consult a qualified health care professional for individual health and medical advice. The author and publisher expressly disclaim any liability, loss, or risk, personal or otherwise, that is incurred as a consequence, direct or indirect, of the use of the application of the contents of this book.

Mention of specific companies, products, organizations or authorities in this book does not imply endorsement by the publisher, nor does it imply that they endorse this book.

Key Porter Books Limited
Six Adelaide Street East, Tenth Floor
Toronto, Ontario
Canada M5C 1H6

www.keyporter.com

Design: Marijke Friesen
Electronic formatting: Jean Lightfoot Peters

Printed and bound in Canada

07 08 09 10 11 6 5 4 3 2 1

TABLE OF CONTENTS

This book is dedicated to all people who have ever struggled with their weight

There is no such thing as a bad body, just bad clothing, bad mirrors and bad diets

MELISSA HERSHBERG

INTRODUCING THE HERSHBERG DIET

What If?

We all know how to lose weight; it's simple, right? We just have to avoid eating carbs, fat, and sugar.

Wait a minute, what about fiber? That's a carb and it's good for weight loss, isn't it? What about the fat content? Should we eat only good fats or avoid fat altogether? What's the glycemic index (GI)? Should we use the GI to guide us and, if so, why isn't the GI value listed on the foods we buy? Some of us think the trick to losing weight is high-protein foods. Some people avoid fat, while others indulge in it so long as the carbohydrate content is low. Some of us read nutrition labels, others don't.

As you can see, despite our years of obsessing over our eating and weight, we don't have a universal and systematic process to use when approaching eating—and it shows. Despite our fixation on weight and the countless fad diets occupying bookstore shelves, approximately one billion people worldwide are considered to be dangerously overweight. According to a Statistics Canada report entitled *Adult Obesity in Canada: Measured Height and Weight* (it can be found at www.statcan.ca/english/research/82-620-MIE/2005001/ articles/adults/aobesity.htm) released in July 2005, approximately 25 percent of Canadian adults are obese and another third are overweight; even more alarming, the numbers are projected to increase unless we put a stop to all this confusion. But wait . . .

What if I revealed that there was a system to correct this problem—a revolutionary weight-loss system that could teach anyone to lose weight and improve their health in just under an hour or two?

What if I told you that the system was based on a unique, never-before revealed combination of three breakthrough nutritional concepts, and so long as you understood these three concepts, you could lose weight easily, quickly, and permanently? Even better, you could lose weight while eating *any* food that you like: fat, carbs, you name it. You could even eat fatty carbs and the weight would still come off. No hunger, no deprivation required.

What if I told you that the system was centered around the discovery of a secret "fourth macronutrient" and that this "fourth macronutrient" is the key to understanding eating for both health and weight loss? Even better, what if I promised that I could prove it to you?

Finally, what if I told you that the system is so easy to implement that it requires no counting grams of fat, protein, or carbohydrates? Would you be intrigued?

Introducing a doctor-designed, breakthrough approach to healthy eating and weight loss! The Hershberg Diet.

The Problem

Before you go on to learn the Hershberg Diet system, I'd like to discuss a growing problem—one more serious than obesity—that has become so prevalent in recent years that medical professionals across the globe now consider it a full-blown epidemic. It is currently estimated that one in four North Americans suffers from this problem; even more alarming, a recent study revealed that 30 to 50 percent of overweight adolescents already have this problem. It plagues men and women, adults and children around the world, as well as the physicians desperate to treat it. So what is it?

The problem is a new medical phenomenon, a type of syndrome that has surfaced in recent years as a direct result of the improper eating habits that have permeated our world. Some call it Syndrome X; others refer to it as the Metabolic Syndrome. I refer to it as, simply, "the Syndrome." Its presence is undeniable; it affects 25 percent of us!

Even if you have not yet heard of the Syndrome, you will. In fact, a large majority of you are already at risk. For instance:

1. Do you have high blood pressure?
2. Do you tend to gain weight around your midsection?
3. Do you seem to constantly struggle with your weight despite eating less than others?
4. Do you suffer from gout?
5. Do you often find yourself wandering back to the fridge or cookie cupboard within only an hour or so of a satisfying meal?
6. Do you suffer from high cholesterol?
7. Are you an adult woman who still struggles with acne, unwanted facial and body hair, and irregular periods?
8. Do you have family members with diabetes?
9. Has your doctor told you that your blood sugar is too high?

10. Do you often skip breakfast, eat a small lunch, and then binge in the evenings?
11. Do you ever feel so hungry that you start to feel sweaty or shaky, and have trouble thinking or concentrating?
12. Do you ever feel high from eating, so much so that you often want to keep eating despite feeling full?

If you answered yes to any of the above questions, you are probably at risk for the Syndrome. In fact, if you answered yes to four of the questions (see below), you may already have the Syndrome.

While not a disease, the Syndrome represents a clustering of risk factors for heart disease, stroke, and cancer. In essence, having the Syndrome means that you have a cluster of disorders related to your metabolism, all occurring at the same time. These disorders include:

- obesity, particularly around the abdomen (i.e., an "apple shape")
- high blood pressure
- abnormal cholesterol (i.e., an elevated level of a blood fat known as triglycerides and a decreased level of the good cholesterol known as HDL)
- insulin resistance (i.e., elevated blood sugar levels).

Having one of the above disorders increases your likelihood of the others; the more components of the Syndrome you have, the greater your risk for heart attack, stroke, diabetes, and certain forms of cancer. Because these afflictions develop in unison, most people who originally see their physician for high blood pressure find out that they also have high cholesterol and are then watched closely for the development of diabetes (high blood sugar). This is how patients progress quickly from being on no medication and requiring relatively few doctor visits to all of a sudden needing to take four daily medications, with the resulting checkups, pill changes, and side effect management and treatment. It's the Syndrome. It's a drug company's dream, a physician's nightmare. And by and large a patient's choice.

You see, unlike other ailments and diseases, the Syndrome is fair. It does not happen by chance, nor does it happen overnight. It happens slowly and predictably with warnings along the way. It offers us a chance to avoid it, reverse it, and beat it. Even better, it offers us a chance to do so drug-free. But we don't.

Study after study has revealed to physicians that the underlying cause of the Syndrome is obesity and improper eating habits. Physicians have known about this diet–health connection for years. After all, it makes sense. Eat too much fat, you'll end up with chronically high levels of fat in the blood (triglycerides). Eat too much sugar, you'll end up with chronically high levels of sugar in the blood (diabetes). The medical literature clearly instructs physicians that the first line of treatment for high blood pressure is diet and exercise. The first line of treatment for high cholesterol is diet and exercise. The first line of treatment for diabetes is diet and exercise. And guess what? The first line of treatment for belly fat is diet and exercise! Obviously, the first line of treatment for the Syndrome is diet and exercise! We know the answer! It's being shouted loud and clear. So why aren't we listening? Why are patients still unaware of this link? Why on earth are we allowing a preventable disease to reach epidemic proportions? More importantly, why have most people still not even heard of the Syndrome?

Some may point to the drug companies. The world's top-grossing drugs treat the components of the Syndrome, so the pharmaceutical companies thrive because of the Syndrome. Most individuals with the Syndrome take at least four medications per day and most often do so for life. Moreover, the pills often cause side effects, which are treated with—you guessed it—more pills. Encouraging diet and exercise is simply bad for business; they work and they're cheap. But the drug companies suffer.

Perhaps it has nothing to do with the drug companies. Maybe the dreaded D&E (diet and exercise) conjures up such thoughts of deprivation, starvation, exhaustion, and misery that people just don't think the sacrifice is worth it. For example, I have heard patients say that living a few years longer is simply not worth giving up the foods they love. I've been told it's about quality of life as opposed to quantity.

And I couldn't agree more. But does life with the Syndrome really allow for higher-quality living that is worth sacrificing longevity? Let's consider what life with the Syndrome is like.

While the Syndrome encompasses a cluster of risk factors for heart attack and stroke, these aren't necessarily how sufferers will die. Remember, the Syndrome attacks slowly, gradually, and progressively. In other words, the Syndrome operates by slowly eating away at the quality of your life. Consider some of the following afflictions that affect people with the Syndrome.

Chronic Kidney Failure

It is estimated that there are roughly one million people worldwide who require dialysis for chronic renal failure (http://bmj.bmjjournals. com/cgi/content/full/327/7413/463). Being on dialysis means spending up to 12 hours per week in the hospital hooked up to a machine—often for the rest of your life. This certainly would reduce quality of life, as frequent symptoms include nausea, fatigue, and loss of appetite. Furthermore, with such a demanding yet necessarily strict schedule, freedom is limited and travel is often no longer possible.

The leading causes of kidney failure are diabetes and high blood pressure.

Limb Amputations

Elevated blood pressure and blood sugar (diabetes) damages blood vessels and nerves. This makes it extremely difficult for the body to heal wounds, even with the help of antibiotics. Often, the only solution to stop the spread of damage is amputation.

More than 60 percent of nontraumatic lower-limb amputations occur among people with diabetes (source is National Diabetes fact sheet 2005—the link is www.diabetes.org/uedocuments/NationalDiabetes FactSheetRev.pdf)

Impotence

Impotence is the inability to obtain or maintain an erection. Although rarely spoken about, impotence is very common among men with the Syndrome. In impotence caused by high blood sugar (diabetes), the nerves that cause an erection may be damaged. In impotence caused by high blood pressure and high cholesterol, the penile artery may be blocked. Impotence can also be the result of medications used to treat high blood pressure. Oh, and by the way, if you have heart disease that requires that you use nitroglycerin to treat angina, as many people with the Syndrome do, Viagra is contraindicated (no longer a safe option). Sorry.

Arthritis

Arthritis, or joint pain, significantly decreases the quality of life of many individuals. It is one of the most common reasons for an elderly individual to visit the doctor. While arthritis results from years of wear and tear on the joints of the hips, knees, and back, for example, the affliction is often experienced earlier and to a more severe degree in individuals with the Syndrome. Why? Well, put simply, years of being overweight translates into years of forcing our joints to sustain that extra weight. This leads to irreversible joint damage for which, unfortunately, aside from total joint replacement, there is often no good treatment or cure.

Cancer

A report from the American Cancer Society reported in *The New England Journal of Medicine*, April 24, 2003, 348, pages 1625–1638—the article is titled "Overweight, Obesity, and Mortality from Cancer"—revealed that in a prospectively studied cohort of U.S. adults, excess body weight and obesity may play a role in a significant number of cancer deaths. The study indicated that 14 percent of cancer deaths in men and 20 percent of cancer deaths in women might be due to being overweight or obese. It was found that the higher the body mass index (weight divided by height squared), the greater the risk of cancer. Among the heaviest participants, the risk of death from cancer was 52 percent higher in men and 62 percent higher in women compared to people of normal weight. Moreover, the data showed that the heaviest men were more likely to die from stomach or prostate cancer, while cancer of the breast, uterus, cervix, or ovary were most likely to cause death among the heaviest women.

The study also indicated that excess weight in the abdomen region (as occurs with the Syndrome) can increase the risk of cancer and that people with obesity may be more likely to develop painful gallstones and acid reflux disease—which can also lead to certain cancers.

Quality of Life

So the "quality of life" argument does not make sense.

The most likely reason that physicians across the globe watch countless patients, young and old, succumb to the Syndrome despite being fully aware of its cause and consequences is because *diet is difficult to prescribe*. While physicians are trained to choose between the countless blood pressure pills, cholesterol pills, and diabetes pills on the market, they are provided with relatively little knowledge on how to choose between the countless diets currently available. For instance, it is unclear whether to counsel patients to eat low-carb or low-fat foods. It is unclear whether to counsel patients about calorie counting and portion control or to simply focus all efforts on teaching about the quality of foods being consumed. The latest literature talks about the glycemic index, but it is time-consuming to rate the glycemic index of individual foods, let alone meals, and, for the most part, most physicians have no idea how to do this. Physicians need a method that is inexpensive and easy to teach, yet offers a prescription that is sensible, easy, and enjoyable for patients and—best of all—will work for life. As you'll soon see, this is the Hershberg Diet.

One of the reasons I entered medicine was to help patients by way of prevention. The practice of medicine was supposed to have shifted in recent years. No longer is it solely about the treatment of symptoms and disease, it's now about health promotion and disease prevention. It's about stopping diseases before they start, as opposed to focusing on treating them once they've already developed. Or so I thought. Yet I found myself watching patient after patient succumb to the Syndrome: a preventable disease! I found myself frustrated and cynical—and I had only just begun. And so I found myself motivated to engender a change. Moreover, I knew that I had the means to do so.

You see, at the age of 15, I virtually stopped eating. My life up until that point had revolved around competitive gymnastics. With a rigorous training schedule of 20+ hours in the gym per week, weight control was never really much of a concern for me. However, when an acute injury abruptly ended my gymnastics career, I found myself gaining weight quickly and unexpectedly. And so I stopped eating. Sure I lost weight—too much weight in fact—but I was miserable and unhealthy. So I began to educate myself about food and nutrition. It was at this point, over 10 years ago, that I discovered what is now the Hershberg Diet system. While I didn't have the scientific or medical knowledge to explain it back then, I knew that it worked, and would work for life. I just didn't know why.

After a science degree and a medical degree, I am happy to report that I now know why. As you will learn in Chapter 1, the explanation rests on the discovery of the "fourth macronutrient." Once I was able to identify this "fourth macronutrient," I was instantly able to articulate and prove the efficacy of the system that I have sworn by for years. I knew that I had discovered a system that could help millions of people lose weight and beat the Syndrome. What I didn't know was how I would convince others that I had the solution. After all, you can imagine the skepticism I encountered—a recent graduate proclaiming to have an innovative diet plan suitable for treating the medical epidemic of the 21st century! Who on earth would believe that?

Well, after being questioned and ridiculed, I was able to convince friends, family, patients, and colleagues. Why? Because the system works—and science and math prove it.

I promise that there is no other dietary system that makes more sense and is easier to understand or follow. This system not only helps you shed weight quickly but also provides a lifelong strategy that will help you maintain your weight and beat the Syndrome.

Overview

I have divided the book into two parts: Part One, The Science, and Part Two, The Hershberg Diet Weight-Loss Plan. In Part One, I introduce and explain three breakthrough nutritional concepts. In Part Two, I'll give you a structured and easy-to-follow four-phase diet plan. It's that simple.

PART ONE: The Science

In Part One, you'll find out about the three breakthrough nutritional concepts that form the basis of the Hershberg Diet. Let's have a peek at them now.

1. **The "fourth macronutrient"** The first and most important concept is how to recognize the "fourth macronutrient." In addition to the three macronutrients with which you may be familiar (fat, protein, and carbohydrate), there is a "fourth macronutrient" to consider. This overlooked and ignored "fourth macronutrient," revealed in Chapter 1, is the key to understanding weight loss. The higher a food is in this "fourth macronutrient," the better it is for weight loss. Once you understand how to identify and factor in this "fourth macronutrient," you will never look at foods, or nutrition labels, in the same way. To lose weight comfortably and quickly, you must learn how to determine which foods are highest in the "fourth macronutrient." These are the foods best for weight loss. As you will see in Chapter 1, this is a mathematical fact and I can prove it!

2. **The "hotty" effect** The second important concept is "hotty" foods. These foods are so named because eating them encourages

the body to heat up and burn calories. "Hotty" foods are difficult for the body to digest and metabolize and, as a result, calories are burned—the body literally heats up as a result. Furthermore, many "hotty" foods and drinks activate hormones that can encourage weight loss. Imagine that! Eating can actually help us lose weight—now, that's hot!

3. **The hormonal effect** The third and final concept that you will learn is how to avoid insulin resistance. In addition to helping prevent cardiovascular disease and diabetes, this knowledge will help you understand why you may be gaining weight despite eating very little. The explanation almost always resides in the body's response to insulin, a hormone released from the pancreas that encourages the storage of fat when handled incorrectly. You will learn that when you overconsume or improperly combine foods that spike blood sugar and insulin, you create a hormonal situation that encourages the body to store fat. You will learn how to train your body to better handle insulin to create a hormonal environment more suited for weight loss.

PART TWO: The Hershberg Diet Weight-Loss Plan

The Hershberg Diet weight-loss plan is divided into four easy phases:

PHASE One Phase One is a two-week initiation phase. It is the strictest phase of the diet. Foods high in the "fourth macronutrient" are emphasized. By the end of this phase, you will notice a significant change in your body: unhealthy high-sugar cravings will be reduced and your body will already begin to look and feel better as fat tissue is lost and water retention decreases.

PHASE Two The next two weeks will constitute Phase Two of the diet plan. This phase is less strict, as you can now include foods that are lower in the "fourth macronutrient." However, these foods still possess the proper "hotty" and hormonal effect, so weight loss will continue as metabolism and fat-burning hormones remain elevated.

PHASE Three Phase Three is the final phase for weight loss. You will remain in this phase until you reach your goal weight. In this phase, you can eat any food you like, although the majority of your diet will still consist of the foods introduced in Phases One and Two. I will show you how you can afford to treat yourself every day and still lose weight while promoting your health.

PHASE Four Phase Four is maintenance. You will remain in this phase for life! The Hershberg Diet system is not a fad diet; it's a healthy lifestyle.

Additional Content

Throughout Phases One and Two, I will include TIPS boxes to highlight additional benefits associated with the foods that you will be eating. For example, you will learn which foods can help attack menstrual cramps and bloating as well as which foods to eat to help prevent prostate and colon cancer. I will show you how drinking the proper drinks and using certain spices can help you speed weight loss and promote your health.

Phases One and Two also include an extensive collection of recipes that are practical, delicious, and easy. For instance, you will learn how to cook the perfect veggie and cheese omelette while brushing your teeth and how to cook a complete dinner of fish and veggies to perfection in just five minutes. I even provide you with recommended brand names for ready-to-eat, store-bought items. No plan could be simpler. On the Hershberg Diet, not having time to eat well is never an excuse!

Phases One, Two, and Three all contain day-by-day sample menu plans. You may follow the plans exactly or simply use them as guides.

My revolutionary approach to eating will change the way you view food. You will feel neither hungry nor deprived. With the Hershberg Diet weight-loss plan, you can eat any, and as much, food as you like, provided that you use the strategies you learn here in this book.

The Hershberg Diet is an easy-to-follow, sensible, and—most of all—enjoyable eating plan.

Let's get started!

PART ONE

THE SCIENCE OF THE HERSHBERG DIET

CHAPTER 1

THE SECRET "FOURTH MACRONUTRIENT"

TRUE OR FALSE?

Q: Despite our obsession with thinness, diet books, and health products, the large majority of us are still completely unaware of the most important and fundamental concept underlying the understanding of nutrition and weight loss.

A: True!

Don't believe me? Consider this:

Almost every medical text, nutritionist, and diet that I have come across states that there are three macronutrients (protein, carbohydrate, and fat) that constitute all food. You have probably heard this before. If you haven't, consider the diets that have been popular in

America over the decades. They are either low-fat (think Susan Powter in the '90s), low-carbohydrate (think Atkins), or low-protein (think poorly constructed vegan/vegetarian diets). We are a society that has altered our fat, carb, and protein ratios for years, yet continues to grow heavier and heavier!

I propose that it is this accepted basic nutritional principle that is responsible for our dietary failures. This flawed principle will continue to hamper even our most valiant weight-loss efforts. Before we can adopt healthy eating habits, lose weight, keep it off, and—most importantly— teach our children how to eat, we must recognize that there are **four** macronutrients.

In this chapter, you will learn how to recognize this "fourth macronutrient" and how to incorporate it into your understanding of food and nutrition labels. As you'll see, it is the single most important factor to consider when deciding how good a food is for weight loss.

Before I open your eyes to this secret "fourth macronutrient," let's quickly review the other three (protein, carbs, and fat), along with some basic nutritional principles. Bear with me while we review the basics; the information that follows will change the way you view food, nutrition labels, and weight loss forever!

The Macronutrients

Protein Proteins comprise mostly carbon, hydrogen, oxygen, and nitrogen atoms. These atoms make up amino acids that link together in various ways to create the variety of proteins found within our bodies (i.e., hair, muscle, nails) and foods. Examples of foods high in protein are meats, fish, poultry, and some legumes. **Proteins contain 4 calories per gram.**

Carbohydrates All carbohydrates consist of carbon, hydrogen, and oxygen atoms linked together to form sugars. Those that consist of one sugar molecule are called simple sugars and include glucose, fructose, and galactose. Those that contain two simple sugars linked together include lactose (milk sugar), sucrose (table sugar), and maltose (malt sugar). Polysaccharides consist of many simple sugars linked together to create starch, cellulose, and glycogen. Polysaccharides are big and complex; for that reason starch is often called a complex carbohydrate. Complex carbohydrates don't dissolve in water like the simple sugars, but rather absorb water. Examples of foods high in carbohydrates are breads, pasta, rice, potatoes, sweets, desserts (like cake, doughnuts, etc.) and candy, milk, fruits, and some veggies. **Carbohydrates contain 4 calories per gram.**

Fat Dietary fats consist mainly of carbon and hydrogen atoms. When they are solid at room temperature, they are called fats; when they are liquid, we call them oils. Saturated fats (e.g., in butter, red meat, cream, cheese, and egg yolk) tend to be from animal sources. Unsaturated fats, either monosaturated or polyunsaturated (i.e., olive oil, vegetable oil, canola oil, nuts, and seeds), tend to be from plant sources. Polyunsaturated fats contain the essential fatty acids, such as omega-6 and omega-3 fatty acids, that we must get from our diet because our bodies cannot make them. Good sources of omega-6 are unrefined corn, sesame, and sunflower oils. Good sources of omega-3 are oily fish like salmon, flaxseed oil, pumpkin seeds, walnuts, and dark green veggies. The third type of fat is trans fat, sometimes called hydrogenated fat, which is usually man-made and found in fatty snack foods like chips and cookies. While unsaturated fats can be good for us, hydrogenated and saturated fats, if overeaten, are associated with an increased risk of heart and blood vessel disease. **Fats contain 9 calories per gram.**

Calories

Dieting trends over the last few decades have avoided acknowledging calories at all costs. The '90s catchphrase "Calories don't make you fat, fat makes you fat" exemplifies the lunacy of this concept. Calories are nothing more than units of energy; they tell us how much a food is worth in terms of energy content. So when we say that a chocolate bar has 300 calories, we are saying that, after digestion and metabolism, our bodies can potentially receive 300 calories worth of energy from that chocolate bar.

What happens if the body doesn't need that energy though? If we consume more calories than we burn off, we will gain weight. This is not a new concept, nor is it refutable. Remember learning about Newton in high school? His first law of thermodynamics says that energy is neither created nor destroyed, it just changes forms. Well, when it comes to nutrition, the energy (calories) contained in a food, if not spent to fuel our bodies, will get stored as fat for later use. If we keep consuming more energy than we need, our fat stores will certainly add up!

Before we go on to see how all of this information comes together on a nutrition label, let's quickly review the main points:

- Fat contains 9 calories of energy per gram.
- Proteins and carbohydrates each contain 4 calories of energy per gram.
- Calories are units of energy.
- If we consume more calories from food than our body burns off, we will gain weight.

Nutrition Labels and the Secret "Fourth Macronutrient"

Let's take a quick example that explains why we need to understand nutrition labels: fat-free turkey from the deli.

(Before I begin, please note that this example, plus the two that I will present in a few moments, may give some life-long math avoiders a bit of a headache! To prove my point that we absolutely must recognize the "fourth macronutrient" if we want to understand weight loss once and for all, I must take you through the mathematical challenges that follow. For many people, this section will be worth the couple of minutes of brainpower required, as it is enlightening. If, however, you choose to just skim it, don't worry. You will not have to do these calculations on the Hershberg Diet weight-loss plan. In fact, I promise you there is no counting of fat grams, carb grams, or protein grams required at all!)

Okay, back to our example. Would you agree that turkey is a protein? Yes. Would you agree that 3 to 4 ounces (100 grams) of fat-free turkey is a reasonable portion size? Yes again. Remember, protein costs 4 calories per gram. So, if we do our calculations, one portion of fat-free turkey should cost 100 grams × 4 calories/gram = 400 calories! Wow, that's a lot of calories; after all, a chocolate bar is only about 300 or so calories. What's going on? How can fat-free turkey, a prototypical diet food, cost more calories than a chocolate bar? The answer is that it doesn't; 100 grams of fat-free turkey provides 100 or so calories. What happened? We better take a closer look at nutrition labels to help us sort out the confusion.

Nutrition labels list a food's serving size as well as its calories, fat, protein, and carbohydrate content. In addition, there's usually a breakdown (in grams) of the different types of carbohydrates found in the food, such as fiber, sugar, and starch. Similarly, the fat content is often organized into different types of fat, such as saturated, monosaturated, and polyunsaturated. All of this adds up to one confusing label!

The nutrient information is based on a specified amount of food. Compare this to the amount you eat.

This number is the amount of the nutrient in the specified quanitity of food.

The Nutrition Facts table will include this list of Calories and 13 nutrients.

Nutrition Facts		
Per 125 mL (87g)		
Amount		**% Daily Value**
Calories 80		
Fat 0.5 g		**1**%
Saturated 0 g + Trans Fat 0 g		**0**%
Cholesterol 0 mg		
Sodium 0 mg		**0**%
Carbohydrate 18 g		**6**%
Fiber 2 g		**8**%
Sugars 2 g		
Protein 3 g		
Vitamin A 2%	Vitamin C 10%	
Calcium 0%	Iron 2%	

The % Daily Value gives a context to the amount of the nutrient in the specified amount of food. The Daily Values are based on recommendations for healthy eating.

The popular fad diets suggest that so much nutritional data is too much information for consumers to comprehend, so they encourage us to focus only on certain parts of a product's nutrition label. Low-fat diets claim that we need pay attention only to the fat grams, low-carbohydrate diets encourage us to look at the carbohydrate content, and cardiologists tell us to pay particular attention to the amount of saturated fat. Clearly, as people are becoming heavier and heavier, this simplified approach is not working.

We must understand the composition of the food that we are eating and look at the entire label. More importantly, we need to recognize that it is what is **not** on the label that matters the most! Let's look at some more examples, keeping in mind that all carbohydrates are 4 calories per gram, all proteins are 4 calories per gram, and all fats are 9 calories per gram. As you'll see, the factor that we should be paying most attention to, the "fourth macronutrient," is not included on the nutrition label at all!

Examples

ROMAINE LETTUCE

Serving size 85 grams

Calories 20

Carbohydrates 3 grams

Protein 1 gram

Fat 0.5 gram

Analysis

3 grams **carb** + 1 gram **protein** + 0.5 gram **fat** = 4.5 grams total

3 g **carb** × 4 cal/g = 12 calories

1 g **protein** × 4 cal/g = 4 calories

0.5 g **fat** × 9 cal/g = 4.5 calories

12 carbohydrate calories +

4 protein calories + 4.5 fat calories = 20.5 calories

3 grams carb + 1 gram protein + 0.5 gram fat = 4.5 grams total

per serving

Nutrition Facts		
Serving Size 6 leaves (85 g)		
Amount For Serving		
Calories 20	Calories from Fat 0	
	% Daily Value*	
Total Fat 0.5 g		**1**%
Saturated Fat 0 g		**0**%
Trans Fat 0 g		
Cholesterol 0 mg		**0**%
Sodium 0 mg		**0**%
Potassium 140 mg		**4**%
Total Carbohydrate 3 g		**1**%
Dietary Fiber 1 g		**4**%
Sugars 2 g		
Protein 1 g		
Vitamin A 20% • Vitamin C 4%		
Calcium 2% • Iron 2%		

*Percent Daily Values are based on a 2,000 calorie diet. Your daily values may be higher or lower depending on your calorie needs.

		Calories:	2,000	2,500
Total Fat	Less than		65 g	80 g
Sat. Fat	Less than		20 g	25 g
Cholestrol	Less than		300 mg	300 mg
Sodium	Less than		2,400 mg	2,400 mg
Potassium			3,500 mg	3,500 mg
Total Carbohydrates			300 g	375 g
Dietary Fiber			25 g	30 g

Calories per gram:
Fat 9 • Carbohydrates 4 • Protein 4

The calories add up almost perfectly. A serving claims to have 20 calories and we have accounted for 20 calories. The grams don't add up at all though. A serving claims to have 85 grams, but we've only accounted for 4.5 grams. What is the nutrition label not telling us?

Let's take another example.

TUNA: GOLDSEAL® SMOKED LIGHT TUNA INFORMATION

(http://www.goldseal.ca/health/nutrient_tuna.asp)

Serving size 55 grams

Calories 60

Carbohydrates 0 grams

Protein 14 grams

Fat 0.2 grams*

* You may be asking yourself: How is there a half gram of fat in romaine lettuce and only a fifth of a gram in tuna? Remember in the section that described fats, where I mentioned that dark green leafy vegetables (like romaine) are good sources of polyunsaturated fat, specifically omega-3 fatty acids? Well this is explains how tuna and romaine compare in fat content—an interesting comparison indeed.

Nutrition Facts Valeur nutritive		
Per ¼ cup (55 g) / par ¼ tasse (55 g)		
Amount **Teneur**	**% Daily Value** **% valeur quotidienne**	
Calories / Calories 60		
Fat / Lipides 0.2 g		1%
Saturated / saturés 0.1 g + Trans / trans 0 g		1%
Cholesterol / Cholestérol 30 mg		
Sodium / Sodium 120 mg		5%
Carbohydrate / Glucides 0 g		0%
Fibre / Fibres 0 g		0%
Sugars / Sucres 0 g		
Protein / Protéines 14 g		
Vitamin A / Vitamine A		0%
Vitamin C / Vitamine C		0%
Calcium / Calcium		4%
Iron / Fer		2%

Analysis

0 grams **carb** × 4 cal/gram = 0 calories

14 grams **protein** × 4 cal/gram = 56 calories

0.2 gram **fat** × 9 cal/gram = 1.8 calories

0 carbohydrate calories + 56 protein calories + 1.8 fat calories = 57.8 calories

0 grams carb + 14 grams protein + 0.2 gram fat = 14.2 grams total per serving

Again, the calories add up almost perfectly. A serving claims to have 60 calories and we've calculated 57.8 calories. The grams are way off though. A serving claims to have 55 grams but we've only accounted for 14.2 grams. What is the nutrition label not telling us? Where are the missing 40.8 grams of food coming from?

If you haven't figured out why our calculations aren't working, don't feel bad. If we factor in just the three macronutrients (carbohydrates, protein, and fat), many nutrition labels will never make sense and consumers will forever be confused.

Now let me enlighten you. Consider a substance that has zero calories per gram. You could add as many grams as you wanted and the calorie count would not change.

Water! Water! Water! Water! Water! Water! Water! Water! Water! Water!

No one ever thinks about the water content of food. This is why people have altered their fat, protein, and carbohydrate ratios for years, yet continue to get heavier and heavier! Water is the "fourth macronutrient" and, as you'll see, it is absolutely imperative that we recognize it as such.

Nutrition labels are becoming more common as companies recognize that consumers are demanding the right to know what is in the food that they are consuming. Yet the constituent that matters most—the "fourth macronutrient"—is omitted. Now that we understand that water constitutes the "fourth macronutrient," we can understand why our calculations didn't add up. You see, 100 grams worth of fat-free deli turkey contains only 100 or so calories because it is mostly water. It has roughly 25 grams of protein at 4 calories per gram (25 grams × 4 calories per gram = 100 calories). The other 75 grams of a 100-gram portion must be zero-calorie water. This makes sense. Think about what happens if you make "turkey jerky." The jerky would weigh much less because all of the water would have evaporated! If we consider that romaine lettuce contains 80.5 grams of water at zero calories per gram, we can see how the calories were correct. The same holds true for tuna with 45.8 grams of water. Similarly, grapefruit, which we consider a carbohydrate, should actually be considered a "water," since the majority of its weight comprises water, hence its low calorie count. If we want to understand weight loss, we must always recognize the "fourth macronutrient." We must learn to *eat* water!

When you eat high-water foods, you get full because you are eating a lot in weight (grams). However, you are consuming a very low number of calories; high-water foods have low energy densities and are therefore the best for weight loss. You can eat them often, and in large portions, and still lose weight. In fact, many high-water foods actually encourage your body to burn calories simply from eating them! We will talk more about this in later chapters. For now, simply remember that the higher a food is in water, the more valuable it is for weight loss.

Now that we understand that water is the "fourth macronutrient," we can start to understand food much better. For instance, why do you think that vegetables "reduce down" so much when you cook them? They are almost entirely water! As you heat them, whether in the wok, oven, or microwave, the water evaporates and you are left with less.

Do an experiment. Take an entire bag of spinach and put it in an empty pot—no water or anything else. Now turn on the heat and stir the spinach a little. What happens? The spinach starts to cook, and although it initially filled the pot, now it doesn't even cover the bottom. Now you can understand why 100 grams of spinach has only about 12 or so calories. It should really be considered a "water," not a carbohydrate. When we eat foods that are high in water, we get a lot of grams for very few calories. Let's look at how the opposite is true as well.

What do people engaged in high levels of activity, such as a long hike or a canoe trip, like to eat? Trail mix! It's a favorite for providing lots of energy, and is therefore high in calories. Now think about what it contains: dried fruit, granola, and nuts. Eating these dry foods allows us to consume loads of calories without getting full. There are no zero-calorie water grams to factor into the amount we are eating. Every bite of that trail mix will be counted as calories. Great for energy, bad for weight loss! Yet many people who don't understand the importance of the "fourth macronutrient" eat these dried foods and believe that they are good for weight loss. Sorry, but unless you are planning to engage in strenuous physical activity, these dried types of foods can lead to rapid weight gain.

Let's Eat How We Want to Be

It astounds me that our society has ignored water as a macronutrient for so long, considering our biology.

People say that we are what we eat, and I couldn't agree more. When we eat diets that are high in fat and sugar, we tend to become overweight (high body fat) and diabetic (high blood sugar). Our bodies literally turn into fat and sugar! I therefore propose that we eat how we want to be—thin and youthful.

The majority—roughly 60 to 70 percent—of our body weight is water. Although water makes up the majority of what we are, the percentage varies with age and body fat. The younger and leaner an individual is, the more water she contains, and vice versa. Consider for a moment why pediatricians stress the importance of fluids when a child is sick. Because children need such a high percentage of body water, they cannot afford to lose water like adults can; they dehydrate easily. Often, hydration status determines whether children will be admitted to hospital when sick. Dehydrated children are fatigued and lethargic with sunken eyes and lax skin. They look aged!

Water is not only crucial for our biological functioning, but also promotes a youthful, healthy appearance. The more high-water foods we consume, the leaner and younger we will feel and appear.

History has provided obvious hints as well. Before food processing, we ate fresh foods: fruits, veggies, milk, meats, seeds, and grains. However, because of the increasing amounts of high-sugar processed foods like candy, pop, cookies, etc., we no longer satisfy our sweet tooth with healthy fruits. Although both contain sugar, factor in the "fourth macronutrient." Candy and fruits both contain simple sugars as their main ingredient on the nutrition label, but fruit is a high-water, high-fiber food. So we can eat an entire apple for the same caloric price as three or so candies. Which choice would make you more "full?" We can consume handfuls of candy or cookies at a sitting because there is no water to fill up our stomach. Our stomachs need a critical weight of food to make us feel "full." Without the water, our stomachs trigger our brain to tell us to eat larger portions to attain the same fullness—and the calories add up.

If you are still unconvinced, close your eyes and picture a typical convenience store. Picture all the goodies that you would consider buying. I am thinking of chips, pretzels, cookies, and even supposedly "healthy" protein bars. Now, notice what all these snack foods have in common. They are dry! They have no free (zero-calorie) water in them. Each time you chew and swallow, you will be consuming calories! Even the protein bars that we think are healthy aren't always! They often have a lot of fat, which is low in water. Fat is hydrophobic, meaning that oil and water don't mix; the fat repels the water. So the more fat a food contains, the less water it will usually contain. Further, fat costs 9 calories per gram; it's pricey! Okay, so what about the high-quality protein contained within these bars, you ask? Well, the protein is in "isolate" form. This means that the water has been taken out! Now you can understand why protein bars are often marketed as meal replacements. They are so low in water that approximately four bites' worth is equivalent in calorie content to an entire meal. Protein bars are densely packed sources of energy (calories). Again, this is great if you are planning on doing rigorous activity, need a meal replacement, or are trying to put on weight. But if you are not, you will likely be taking in more energy that your body needs. As we have learned, the leftover calories will simply be stored as fat!

It is no coincidence that as our world has become more convenient, our food has become drier, and we have become heavier. We must look back to correct our dietary mistakes.

Chapter Summary

- Water is the "fourth macronutrient" that is essential to weight loss.
- Water has zero calories per gram.
- The more water a food contains, the better it is for weight loss.

How Fancy Marketing Tricks May Be Making You Fat

Ever heard of low-carb beer or zero-carb rum? I'm sure you have. Almost all alcohol is now marketed as low-carb. Take Bacardi's recent advertising for Bacardi White: zero sugar, zero carbs, 66 calories. Sounds great, doesn't it? Let's put this marketing to the test.

Based on what I've explained so far, there are three basic macronutrients: carbs, protein, and fat. However, as we've seen, there really should be four. Water is the fourth macronutrient; it is an essential part of food and contributes to its weight. When we analyze a nutrition label, we must consider how each of the macronutrients is contributing to the food's overall nutritional content. The same theory must be applied to drinks.

If Bacardi White has zero carbs, then where on earth do the 66 calories come from? It isn't protein. It isn't fat—alcohol is fat-free. So where are the calories coming from? If there are no carbs, as the advertisement promises, and no protein nor fat, then it must be the fourth macronutrient, water. But this makes no sense. Water does not get us drunk and, furthermore, water has zero calories.

Stumped? I bet you are. You see, even though I just told you that there are three basic macronutrients, and a fourth, water, that contribute to the weight of food, there's actually one more. Alcohol itself! Alcohol is a type of macronutrient. It has 7 calories per gram. To recap,

- Carbohydrates have 4 calories per gram.
- Protein has 4 calories per gram.
- Fat has 9 calories per gram.
- Water has 0 calories per gram.
- Alcohol has 7 calories per gram.

So what exactly is alcohol?

Alcohol is a type of carbohydrate that has been fermented. It contains substances such as fruit, wheat, potato, or barley. Wine is made from grapes. Beer is made from barley. Vodka uses wheat or potato. Grapes, barley, wheat, and potato are carbs. But for these carbs to turn into alcohol, they must be fermented. After fermentation, the carbohydrate is no longer classified as a carb but rather as an alcohol. So, for instance, when barley is in its natural state, it is a carbohydrate and therefore has 4 calories per gram. However, once it has been fermented, it is considered an alcohol and now contains 7 calories per gram. So alcohol is simply a more caloric type of carbohydrate!

This then raises the question, is low-carb beer actually more caloric than full-carb beer? What do you think?

I'll let you ponder this question for a few moments. Before I answer, though, I'd like to tackle alcoholic spirits.

Pure alcoholic spirits such as rum, gin, vodka, or tequila all have zero carbs because they are distilled. The distilling process ensures that all of the carbohydrate (e.g., the wheat or potato) has been fermented to alcohol, leaving no carbs behind.

So based on what I've taught, can you guess how many calories 1 ounce of vodka contains?

Well, 1 ounce is equivalent in weight to 28 grams. So if alcohol contains 7 calories per gram and there are zero carbs, zero protein, and zero fat, then we may reasonably conclude that 1 ounce (28 grams) of vodka would contain 196 calories, (28 grams × 7 calories per gram = 196).

This seems like a lot doesn't it? Well, of course it does. Remember, vodka isn't 100 percent alcohol; it's more like 50 percent alcohol. So this means that the rest, the other 50 percent, is water. So a 1-ounce (28 gram) serving of vodka contains approximately 14 grams of alcohol (14 grams × 7 calories per gram = 98 calories) and 14 grams of water (14 grams × 0 calories per gram = 0 calories). This makes sense. One shot of vodka is approximately 100 calories.

So now that we understand spirits, let's get back to the beer brain-buster.

If carbohydrates contain 4 calories per gram and alcohol contains 7 calories per gram, is low-carb beer more caloric than full-carb beer?

The answer is yes, sometimes. In order to understand this, we must review how beer is made.

Unlike hard alcohol, beer is not fully distilled. While the majority of the carbohydrate, barley, for example, is fermented to alcohol, some of it remains in carbohydrate form. This is why beer doesn't taste as strong as hard alcohol; it's sweeter and more filling. And this explains why many people have difficulty putting back straight vodka yet have no problem putting back straight beer. Beer contains three macronutrients: alcohol, carbohydrate, and water.

To get a low-carb beer, one of the following two things has to happen:

1. The water content must be increased. If we keep the same size can of beer but make it higher in water, the alcohol and carb content remaining will naturally decrease. This trick has been known for a long time and is the recipe for many light beers. Coors Light, for instance, is lower in carbs than regular beer because it has more water and therefore less carbohydrates and less alcohol. A bottle of light beer makes us less tipsy than a bottle of regular beer (because the former has less alcohol) and tastes lighter (because it has less carbohydrate and more water). Light beer is less caloric than traditional beer because it has more water; and water has zero calories.

2. The leftover carb content must be decreased. When the low-carb era began, beer companies jumped on the bandwagon and came up with a new way of making beer. The new method of "mashing" carbs allows more of the carbs to be fermented to alcohol. These low-carb beers therefore often lack the flavor and body of regular beers. And guess what? They are more caloric because alcohol has nearly double the calories as regular carbohydrates, gram for gram.

Committed low-carb dieters have become so brain-washed by fancy marketing that they have forgotten the reason Dr. Atkins, the guru himself, swore off carbs in the first place. He blamed carbohydrates for today's obesity epidemic because carbs spike insulin levels. And, as you'll learn in Chapter 3, insulin is a fat-storing hormone.

On the Atkins diet, carbs are considered the enemy whereas fat and protein are encouraged because they are LESS likely to cause you to store fat. While there is some merit to this theory, the majority of low-carb dieters have completely missed the point. The advertising of alcohol as carb free or low carb exemplifies this point.

Alcohol raises insulin even more than carbohydrates! When we ingest alcohol, we absorb it into our blood very quickly. After all, as we've learned, alcohol is nothing more than fermented carbohydrates, and fermented carbohydrates raise insulin just like natural carbohydrates.

So alcohol is more caloric than carbohydrates and spikes our fat-storing insulin hormone as well. So who cares that alcohol is low in carbs? It would actually be better for us if it had more carbs and less alcohol: it'd be much better for us to eat straight barley (a fibrous complex carb) than fermented barley (an alcohol).

But for those—like me—who are not willing to forgo alcohol for life, don't worry. In Part Two, I have included a section on alcohol to show you how you can drink it while still losing weight and maintaining your health.

CHAPTER 2

THE "HOTTY" EFFECT

The second important concept when it comes to weight loss is "hotty" foods. "Hotty" foods are so named because eating them encourages the body to heat up because calories are being burned! When we burn calories, heat is released. Read this again.

You see, simply by eating certain foods, you encourage your body to burn calories. This is because some foods are harder to digest and metabolize than others and, as a result, calories are burned. Consider eating these foods as exercise for your digestive tract! Before I go on to discuss what makes food "hotty," let's take a minute to discuss the concept of calorie burning.

Every time your body works to heat itself up, you are burning calories. The more heat you make, the more calories you have burned. So an easy way to understand calorie burning and weight loss is to think about some of the things in life that cause us to heat up! Let's look at some of these now. (And no, putting on a jacket does not count!)

Exercise Exercise is certainly the most obvious thing that comes to mind. Think of what happens when we go for a jog or a bicycle ride, for instance. We heat up and start to sweat. Ever wonder why?

When we exercise, our bodies convert a stored form of energy into a form of energy that we can use for fuel. During this energy conversion, heat is released. Because we need to keep a constant body temperature, we quickly rid ourselves of this excess heat by sweating. As the perspiration evaporates, it cools us. So even though we're producing heat, our sweat glands protect us from overheating. Why is this important for weight loss? Well, the majority of energy is stored in the body as fat! It makes sense, then, that the more heat we produce, the more fat we burn! Actually, this is how metabolism can be measured. People are placed in water and those who create the most heat, causing the water to heat up the most, are said to have the fastest metabolism. The faster a person's metabolism is, the quicker she can convert fat into fuel and the more heat she produces in doing so. This is why people with fast metabolisms have an easier time staying thin.

So aside from giving you another reason to detest these fast-metabolizing skinny minnies, why should you care about this? Well, by understanding this concept, you can appreciate why exercise is so important for health and weight loss. Exercise increases metabolism and causes you to convert stored energy (fat) into usable energy (fuel). Now that you know that heat is the byproduct, you can't deny that exercise is critical for weight loss. Nothing causes you to sweat more, and therefore there is nothing better for burning calories, period. The next time you break a sweat, the next time you feel the "burn," you know your effort will be rewarded by calories burned!

Any diet plan that says that exercise is not important is bogus. The more exercise you do, the more calories you will burn. You must get active to expedite weight loss! It doesn't matter what you do as long as you work up a sweat!

Resting metabolism Human beings are homeotherms. This means that humans try to maintain a constant body temperature, about 98.6°F (37°C), at all times no matter what their environment. This is why we feel sick when we have a fever. Our body temperature is not meant to go above this set point, so we feel shivery, sick, and unwell. So how does the body keep this constant temperature? Well, one way is via our resting metabolism. Even when we aren't exercising, our bodies are converting food energy (the calories we consume from the food we eat) and/or stored energy (the calories of energy that are stored on our body as glycogen or fat) into usable energy (fuel) and the byproduct is heat. We don't feel sweaty at rest like we do when we exercise because we are doing this at a much slower rate and we need much less fuel when we are at rest. Sure, our heart still has to beat, our lungs have to breathe, our cells have to repair, but this is relatively easy compared to the mega work we have to do when running or biking. So how can we force our bodies to work harder and therefore burn more calories when we are at rest? By having more lean muscle tissue.

Muscle cells take a lot of work to maintain compared to the other cells in the body. This means that two people who weigh the same amount, who eat the same amount of food, and who both choose to laze around for the day doing nothing will burn a different number of calories depending on how much of their weight is made up of muscle. The 180-pound sprinter who is mostly muscle is a calorie-burning machine, whereas the 180-pound professional TV watcher who is mostly fat is burning very few calories. So what happens? The athlete gets thinner and the couch potato gets heavier, even though they're both sitting around doing nothing and eating the same amount of food! So the moral is that we must weight train and increase our muscle mass if we want to speed up our resting metabolism and burn more calories at rest. The best part is that after a session of weight training, our metabolism stays elevated because our muscles must work to repair themselves—burning even more calories!

Hormones Picture this: you hate public speaking. It's your brother's wedding and he's asked you to speak. You're up next. You're freaking out. Your heart is pounding. You can barely catch your breath. Your mouth feels dry. Your face is flushed. You're heating up. You're sweating buckets. Help! Is this familiar? Even if you love an audience and relish the opportunity to speak in public, everyone is stressed out by something, whether it is asking someone out on a date or getting caught in a lie. We've all felt these physical reactions and they manifest in the same ways for all of us. This is our fight-or-flight response, and it is triggered when we sense a potential threat. It's our sympathetic nervous system hormones—mainly adrenaline and its relative, noradrenaline—creating the physical reactions.

So why is this important when it comes to weight loss? Well, did you notice that part of this reaction involved sweating? These hormones can be thought of as fat-melting hormones. They are great at creating heat and burning calories! And while these hormones help us in times of stress, they're bad for us if released too often. However, there are ways to gently activate these hormones, thereby encouraging the body to burn calories without the negative consequences. The first is exercise. The second, however, is not as obvious: there are foods and drinks that can help us burn a few extra calories via this mechanism. You will learn about these in Phase One of the Hershberg Diet weight-loss plan.

Okay, so now that we understand how different methods of heating up can help us lose weight, let's look at one final way that our body is encouraged to burn calories: the thermogenic effect of food.

Thermogenic effect of food "Thermo" means heat, as in a thermos or thermostat. "Genic" means creating, as in genesis. So "thermogenic" means heat-creating. The more heat we create after eating food, the more calories we burn off and the fewer we have available to store as fat! Some foods are very thermogenic, whereas others are not. By simply eating the right thermogenic foods, then, we can increase our metabolism and burn calories just by eating! From now on, I will refer to these calorie-burning, thermogenic foods as "hotty" foods.

Of the three basic macronutrients, protein is the most "hotty," followed by carbohydrates (complex carbs more so than simple carbs) and then, finally, fats. This means that our body must burn more calories to digest a high-protein meal than either a high-carb meal or a high-fat meal. Why? Well, proteins are big and complex molecules. The body must break these complex molecules down into simpler ones called amino acids before we can absorb and use them. This is hard work. So, when we eat [high-protein foods, such as turkey, chicken, fish, and seafood, for example] we burn calories, thus releasing heat. Protein is "hotty!"

Complex fibrous carbohydrates are the next best at burning calories. Remember from Chapter 1 that the more sugar molecules that are linked together to form a carbohydrate, the more complex the carbohydrate is said to be? We must break down all carbohydrates to glucose (sugar) before the body can absorb and use them. Knowing this, it makes sense that complex carbs are more "hotty" than simple carbs; it takes more work to break them down to glucose and therefore burns more calories in the process. Complex high-fiber carbohydrates (like whole wheat bread, brown rice, and oatmeal, for example) are like complex literature: it takes a long time to digest the material, but once you do, the effort is rewarded! Complex high-fiber carbs are "hotty!"

Simple and low-fiber carbs (like candy and processed refined snack foods—chips, cookies, pretzels, white bread, white rice, and sugary cereals, for example) are simple to digest and, as a result, the work is not as rewarded by calories burned. Simple and low-fiber carbs are therefore not "hotty."

Fat is the least "hotty" of the basic macronutrients. Before fat can enter our bloodstream, it must be digested to fatty acids and glycerol.

As you may have guessed, this is done easily and few calories are burned as a result. But there's a catch. The process is also done quite slowly. Although we aren't burning very many calories, we are staying quite full because it takes a long time for the digestive process to complete. Fats therefore fill us up. When we eat fat along with the other macronutrients, it can actually help us by slowing the rate at which the whole meal is absorbed. So while fat is the least "hotty," don't cut it out of your diet just yet.

On the Hershberg Diet plan, I will show you which foods to eat and how to eat them so that you capitalize on all these pros while avoiding the cons.

Let's review what we have learned so far:

- Get active to burn calories. Breaking a sweat means burning calories. That's why you feel hot when you exercise!
- Build muscle to speed up resting metabolism. Maintaining a muscle cell is harder work than for any other cell and, as a result, calories are burned. The more muscle you have, the more calories you will burn at rest. You will also burn extra calories following a session of weight training because your body is still working hard to build and repair the muscle fibers. If you feel the burn, smile, because you're burning calories!
- Activating the right hormones can help you burn calories. You will learn more about this in the next chapter. You will also learn which foods to eat to gently stimulate these hormones.
- In terms of calorie-burning "hotty" foods, protein are the most "hotty," then complex high-fiber carbs then low-fiber simple carbs then fat.

Okay, let's go on to Chapter 3. Once you complete this final introductory chapter, you are ready for The Hershberg Diet weight-loss plan.

THE HORMONAL EFFECT

Now that we understand how the "fourth macronutrient" (water) and thermogenesis ("hotty" foods) contribute to weight loss, we are ready to tackle the third and final concept—the hormonal effect.

In this chapter, you will learn how to create the optimal hormonal environment for weight loss. In addition to helping prevent cardiovascular disease and diabetes, the information you will learn will help you understand why you may be gaining weight despite eating very little food. The explanation almost always resides in the body's response to insulin.

So what is insulin?

Insulin is a hormone made by the pancreas. It is an incredibly important hormone as, without it, we could not live. Insulin allows sugar (remember, all carbohydrates are digested to sugar) to move from our bloodstreams into our cells. Once the sugar enters our cells, it undergoes a process called cellular respiration in order to make fuel ("cellular" because it's in our cells, and "respiration" because it requires that we breathe in oxygen and breathe out carbon dioxide). Without this fuel, we could not function; we would be like a car without gas. So insulin is a very important hormone. But insulin also signals the body to store fat, a process called lipogenesis. You see, sugar can easily be converted to fat instead of fuel. Why? Well, think of your body as a car again.

What do you do when your car's gas gauge approaches empty? You start to look for the nearest gas station for a fill-up, right? Well, when the fuel in the body runs low, the body starts to think about how it will get its next fill-up. Of course, we could eat food, but in the past, food was not always readily available. We had to be able to have a backup method, and we do. Remember from last chapter that we have energy stored on the body that is capable of making fuel. Energy is stored on our hips, thighs, bellies, etc. as fat, and it's also stored in the muscle and liver as glycogen, a type of carbohydrate. Like food, the fat on the body contains about 9 calories of energy per gram and the carbohydrate (glycogen) in the muscle and liver has about 4 calories of energy per gram. So if we can't eat to fill up, we simply break down these stores and release the energy. Insulin is the hormone that allows us to store energy (fat) on the body for later use.

When we eat a meal, we use some of the sugar (remember, all carbohydrates break down to sugar) for fuel, but if we have some left over, we store it for later. The insulin allows the sugar to get into all of our cells and, if it's not used right away for fuel, it will be converted to glycogen or fat and stored for later use.

Certain foods cause sugar to move into our bloodstreams too quickly. Then lots of insulin is released and some fuel is made—but there is a lot of leftover sugar to deal with. We get a sugar spike followed by an insulin spike followed by fat deposition followed by a crash in blood sugar. Now the situation worsens. When blood sugar levels are low, our brain thinks that we are starving; that we need more food, more sugar. So we incorrectly feel hungry and then seek out more food...more food that we'll simply store as fat! We feel hungry but for the wrong reason. We don't need more fuel; we have incorrectly caused our blood sugar levels to plummet because we ate unnatural sugar-spiking foods.

When we overeat sugar-spiking foods, we over-release insulin and we store too much fat. But the body is smart; it tries to protect us from overeating by rejecting the insulin! This is how insulin resistance, the precursor to diabetes, develops. **FYI**, if your doctor has told you that you are "pre-diabetic" or have "insulin resistance," this is likely what's happening within your body. At this stage, if you start watching your eating and changing your food habits, the situation may be reversible. However, this is not what the majority of us do.

When we don't change our eating habits, we force the pancreas to give us more insulin. We encounter a situation called hyperinsulinemia (high insulin levels in the blood), which is how the body tries to beat the insulin resistance. And it works—for a little while. The problem is that now we are en route to becoming significantly overweight and diabetic. Let's look at why.

Although we have more insulin around, it doesn't work nearly as well as it used to. So some sugar stays trapped in our blood, unable to enter our cells. This is why we start to develop chronically high blood sugar levels irrespective of whether we've eaten. **FYI**, this is the reason that doctors order *fasting* blood work; they want to see how high your blood sugar level is when you haven't eaten. If your blood sugar is high, the doctor knows that the hormonal situation in your body is not optimal. Even worse, these chronically high blood sugar levels trick the pancreas into thinking that we need even more insulin. Remember, it is insulin's job to clear the sugar from the blood by allowing it to enter our cells. So now, with insulin not working properly, we always have high blood sugar levels, we always want more insulin to help clear them, and we are always in a state of telling our bodies to store fat, even when we haven't eaten! Believe it or not, the situation gets even worse.

For fat loss to occur, the body likes insulin levels to be low. When insulin levels are low, the body thinks that blood sugar must be getting too low, and if blood sugar is low, the body quickly uses its fat and glycogen stores to make fuel. So low insulin levels are associated with fat loss. When insulin levels are low, certain special hormones (including the adrenaline and noradrenaline discussed in Chapter 2) are signaled to fire. These hormones signal our body fat stores to turn into fuel and heat.

People often think that overweight people who claim to be dieting and not losing weight are lying. How can they be consuming so little and not losing weight? Now you know how! Having eaten too many of the wrong sugar-spiking foods in the past, they created a situation of chronically high blood sugar and insulin. As a result, the body is constantly in a state of thinking that it must either need to make fuel or store fat, because why else would sugar and insulin levels be high? You see, overeating sugar-spiking foods creates a situation whereby you gain weight easily even when you're not eating very much. It's like going further and further into debt even when you're not spending money—simply because the interest is accumulating.

To add insult to injury, the chronically high insulin levels discourage fat-melting hormones from firing! It is no wonder that the ambitious dieter is not losing weight. How could he when his body is in a constant state of wanting to accumulate fat and not wanting to burn it?

It is at this point that family doctors often detect early diabetes. Through screening of urine or blood, a high sugar level is found. The first line of treatment is diet; unfortunately, people are often not told that it must be a diet that discourages blood sugar and insulin levels from spiking. It must be a diet that recruits the fat-burning hormones. It must be a diet that prevents metabolism from slowing. Finally, it must be a diet that is filling, palatable, nutritious, and sustainable.

The Hershberg Diet weight-loss plan meets all of these criteria. It is easy to follow and medically sound. The foods that are promoted help stabilize insulin and blood sugar levels. Through eating these foods, nutrients will be absorbed slowly into the bloodstream. This controlled release will prevent blood sugar and insulin spikes. Fat-burning hormones will be activated not only through this lowering of insulin levels but also by the use of "hotty" foods. "Hotty" foods can gently stimulate these fat-melting hormones, adding additional ammunition for your fat-loss goal. The diet is sustainable; you are encouraged to eat foods from all of the macronutrient categories and even allowed to indulge any of your cravings, provided that you follow the techniques taught in the next section. It is through these healthy eating habits that we will win the fight against obesity, insulin resistance, and diabetes and beat the Syndrome once and for all.

Let's review the major concepts introduced in this section:

- Insulin promotes sugar uptake into cells and its conversion to fuel and heat, with leftovers being stored largely as fat.
- High insulin levels can cause us to accumulate fat easily, even when we haven't eaten!
- Foods that spike blood sugar and insulin levels encourage the situation of fat storage as opposed to fat melting.
- Chronically high blood sugar and insulin levels discourage the release of fat-melting hormones.
- Eating foods that prevent spikes in blood sugar and insulin levels will help create an optimal environment for weight loss.

Fad Diets Analyzed

We live in a fast-paced world. We crave immediacy, high speed, and instantaneous results. We want instant oatmeal, instant rice, immediate service, and fast food. We want high-speed Internet banking, automatic tellers, and instant wealth. While we seek speedy results when it comes to both our weight and our wealth, we use better judgment when it comes to the latter. Whereas we are skeptical of get-rich-quick schemes, we fall for fad diet after fad diet, without ever taking the time to question the underlying rationales.

As you'll see, many popular fad diets are founded on flawed science. While they may work for the short term, their restrictive nature often makes them unsustainable. More importantly, their flawed reasoning can set us up for weight gain and at times even harm our health. Let's take a closer look at these dietary "get-rich-quick schemes."

Low-Fat Diet

When an entire category of macronutrient is severely restricted from our diets, the result will initially and intuitively be calorie reduction and thus weight loss, unless a substitute is introduced.

Low-fat eating sounds like a nutritionally sound and appropriate solution to the emerging obesity problem. At 9 calories per gram, fat costs twice as many calories as either protein or carbohydrates. Remember from Chapter 1 that fat is hydrophobic, meaning that what you see is what you get in terms of portion (there are no zero-calorie water grams to expand the portion). Ten grams of oil is therefore 90 calories (10 grams × 9 calories per gram = 90 calories). A very low-fat diet certainly seems reasonable because by cutting out fat, we'd be cutting out the most caloric part of our diets. Also, as most snack foods, baked goods, and protein and dairy products contain fat, our food options would be seriously limited. We would have to rely on lean meats, fish, fruits, veggies, potatoes, pasta, rice, and breads. Sounds good, right? Well, let's look at what happens.

Because all types of fat are condemned on low-fat diets, cooking meats and fish becomes challenging. So people on these diets tend to eat foods that are very high in carbohydrates, low in protein, and low in fat. As we've seen, these type of foods, like bagels, crackers, and cereals, are almost purely dry carbohydrate (i.e., they contain virtually no water). As a result, they are not very filling, and it is easy to eat much more than the recommended single portion size (half a bagel, four crackers, one slice of bread, etc.) without feeling full. Further, because these foods are labeled "fat-free" and thus incorrectly interpreted as "calorie-free" by the majority of the population, people eat gargantuan portion sizes, thereby defying the initial plan of cutting calories.

As the low-fat craze caught on, the market became saturated with reduced-fat and fat-free foods. Food scientists teamed with corporate America to remove fat from foods and replace it with the next tastiest thing—

sugar! Now people were loading up on reduced-fat cookies, chips, cakes, ice creams, etc. Although the low-fat replacements were slightly lower in calories than their original forms because sugar has 4 calories to fat's 9 calories per gram, people were more than making up for this difference by increasing portion sizes, thinking that only the fat grams mattered. The prevailing sentiment of the time was, "Calories don't make you fat, fat makes you fat." Unfortunately, as many of us know, this thinking proved dead wrong.

As many of you ex-low-fat dieters know, the result of the low-fat craze for many people was weight gain! People consumed excess calories in the form of fat-free carbohydrates (bagels, candy, rice cakes) and gained weight. Even worse, as most of these high-carb, low-fat foods are dry, with little water weight to expand their volume, people were packing on the pounds while still feeling hungry! Insulin levels surged, stimulating appetite, and the low water content didn't fill us up. Fortunately, people started to wise up and say goodbye to fat-free eating. However, it was only a matter of time before history repeated itself—low-carb America was born.

Very Low-Carbohydrate Diet

Low-carb diets are not new and actually work a lot like the "carb-loading" that marathon runners used to do before a big race. The two sound like opposites, but they're not.

Before a big race, marathon runners would often deplete their carbohydrate stores by eating only fat and protein—think steak, cheese, eggs—a week before the

THE HORMONAL EFFECT 55

race. By eliminating carbs from the diet, the dedicated runner forced his body to draw upon its stored form of carbohydrate—glycogen. (Recall from Chapter 3 that glycogen is a type of carbohydrate that we keep stored in our liver and muscles for emergency energy purposes. This way, when blood sugar or energy is too low, as occurs when we avoid eating carbs, we can quickly convert glycogen into glucose (sugar) and continue functioning.) Now glycogen, like all carbs, is hydrophilic ("hydro" = water; "philic" = loving). This means that it is attracted to water and absorbs it. So the carb-starved athlete would go into a state of glycogen depletion and, for each gram of glycogen lost from his muscle, he'd lose approximately 3 grams of body water along with it. The result was a strategically shrunken, dehydrated body perfectly prepped to rapidly increase in size when the athlete began carb-loading.

You see, a few days before the big race, the athlete would load up on high-carb foods such as pasta and bread. The hungry muscles would get very excited that carbohydrates were once again available, so they would eat them up very efficiently. The glycogen and water were replaced quickly and efficiently, and the runner's muscles could now serve as big, bulky, volume-expanded energy reserves capable of sustaining his energy needs throughout the race.

Most athletes have stopped doing this, though, because the quick water gain was painful to their muscles. In fact, the quick increase in water made it more difficult for the oxygen in the blood to get to the muscle cells. Without oxygen, our cells can make only lactic acid. Increased lactic acid and decreased fuel leads to burning pain and, ultimately, cell death. The scariest part is that this can occur in the heart muscle as well. When a heart doesn't get enough oxygen, this is a heart attack. Now let's see how this is similar to the very low-carbohydrate diet.

In the induction phase of low-carb diets, most carbo-hydrates are severely restricted, even healthy and "hotty" ones like complex carbohydrates, fruits, and most veg-gies. This carbohydrate depletion scares the body into rapidly converting the stored glycogen in the liver and muscle into glucose. Remember, this shrinks the size of the muscles because water is lost with the glycogen. So the satisfying visible weight loss seen at the beginning of these diets is actually mostly water weight!

Once glycogen is used up, the body is forced to use fat and protein sources to make sugar and ketones, an alternative source of fuel. The body is now in "ketosis," which can be very dangerous, especially when combined with dehydration. Thankfully, this potentially dangerous ketotic state is very difficult to sustain. After all, it requires that you stick quite rigidly to a very low-carbohydrate diet.

How many people do you know who have stuck with an extremely low-carbohydrate diet? Not many. It's hard to fight our biochemistry. Often, people stick with it for a month or so. They lose fat, probably about 1 to 2 pounds per week as they are restricting their calories. After all, it's hard not to lose weight when you are restricting an entire macronutrient category (carbohydrates), especially the one that constitutes most snack foods, desserts, and sweets. In addition, people on very low-carb diets lose water, muscle, and bone weight. Delighted with their impressive weight loss, they loosen their restriction and indulge in carbohydrates. Just like the carb-loader marathon runner whose muscles were initially starved, the body now becomes superefficient at storing any consumed sugars. The result: rapid, excessive, and potentially dangerous bloating and weight gain, if muscle cells can't get enough oxygen. If you recall the example of the carb-loader marathon runner I gave earlier, you'll remember that when muscles quickly increase in size from the replacement of glycogen and water, it makes it difficult for the cells to get enough oxygen. And without oxygen, cells die. In the heart muscle, for example, this is called a heart attack or myocardial (heart muscle) infarction (death due to lack of oxygen). So most people regain the weight quickly, only to set themselves up for an even more challenging weight loss the next time around. (Each time we lose weight quickly and then gain it back, we lose lean muscle weight and replace it with fat because it's easier to rebuild fat stores than muscles. As we know from Chapter 2, muscle burns more calories than fat, so the result is less lean muscle tissue, more fat, and slower metabolisms.)

Have you ever heard of a "fat skinny" person? Are you a "fat skinny" person? "Fat skinnies" are created through this process of repeated fad dieting and are people who may not weigh much because they have less muscle, water, and bone weight, but they have high percentages of body fat. "Fat skinnies" may be a size 4, but they don't look nearly as good as a size 4 made of lean muscle tissue and water, and they certainly aren't as healthy. It is perpetual yo-yo dieting that sets people up to become "fat skinnies."

Cyclic weight loss and gain isn't the only problem with these diets. In addition, by eliminating carbohydrates, we deprive ourselves of some very healthy and "hotty" foods: fiber, for instance. Although most green veggies are permitted on low-carb diets, fruit and grain sources of fiber are limited, which increases our risk of constipation, bowel disorders, and some cancers. Also, we miss out on the calorie-burning potential of these foods. Remember from Chapter 2 that breaking down complex fibrous carbohydrates burns a lot of calories as heat. Further, when our bodies digest high-water fibrous carbohydrates, sugars are released into the blood in a controlled fashion. This prevents us from having to break down our muscle and tissue proteins for fuel. As you can see, there are serious problems associated with very low-carbohydrate diets.

Although very low-carbohydrate diets are flawed, we can still learn from them. These diets unintentionally promote the water properties of food. By virtually eliminating one of the three macronutrients from the diet, we are theoretically left with only two-thirds the amount of choice (protein and fat). Once you remove the carbohydrate-rich foods, you are left with meat, fish, and some dairy, fruit, and veggies. Essentially, high-water foods!

You see, the secret to the real and lasting weight loss is not carb deprivation but, rather, committing to a diet of high-water foods!

The Glycemic Index (GI)

This concept has caught on quickly and is now being used widely by medical professionals to counsel their patients on healthy eating. Typically, patients are told that eating a diet of low-GI foods will help prevent diabetes and help them lose weight; they are then sent off to figure out what on earth this means and how they can use it to select healthy foods.

The obsession with a food's GI comes from advances in knowledge of insulin and its effect on hunger, weight, and energy levels as well as the unavoidable reality that we are being faced with an epidemic of diabetes. So what is the GI?

The GI is a ranking of carbohydrates on a scale from zero to 100 according to the rate at which they raise blood sugar levels after eating. Specifically, the GI of a food is assessed by comparing 50 grams of the digestible available carbohydrate component of that food with 50 grams of glucose (a very simple sugar) to see how similar they act in terms of raising blood sugar levels. The closer the food acts to glucose, the higher its GI rating will be and the worse for you it is considered to be. So foods with a high GI, like candy and white bread, quickly raise blood sugar levels whereas foods with a low GI, like oatmeal, raise blood sugar levels more slowly. While this theory certainly sounds scientific and meritorious, let's see how it stands up to closer analysis.

To fully understand the GI, we must first look at what is meant by the phrase "digestible carbohydrate." Not all carbohydrates are digestible. Fiber is defined as an indigestible carbohydrate because it passes through the stomach and intestines without being digested; it provides bulk and therefore helps us stay regular. So because the GI of a food is assessed by comparing 50 grams of the digestible available carbohydrate component of that food with 50 grams of glucose, we must subtract the fat, protein, water, and fiber content of the food to arrive at the actual digestible carbohydrate component leftover. (Remember that fat, protein, water, and fiber aren't digestible carbohydrates—only carbohydrates are carbohydrates.) Are you still with me? This is where the flaws inherent with using the GI system become apparent.

When we eat meals, we do not subtract the protein, fat, fiber, and water content of the food and select portion sizes based on how much digestible carbohydrate is left over. The GI, while useful in theory, does not make sense when it comes to actual eating in real life. Let's take eating an apple as an example.

To arrive at the correct GI of an apple, we'd have to peel it (take out the fiber), then dehydrate it (take out the water), and then eat 50 grams of what's left over to get at the digestible carbohydrate component and therefore the proper GI. Is this how the majority of us eat apples? NO! We bite into them through their peels and enjoy their watery/juicy goodness. Because we're consuming the fiber and the water, we're actually eating less than "50 grams of digestible carbohydrate," so more than one apple must be eaten to arrive at the correct GI value.

Next, let's look at carrots. As some of you may know, carrots have received a bad rap in recent years. Both the Atkins and South Beach diets consider them to be too high in carbs to be eaten regularly when trying to lose weight. And now even the health-conscious GI dieters are avoiding this veggie as it has been rated as a very high-GI food. But based on what I have just taught, this just isn't the case.

Carrots are high in fiber and water, and are difficult to consume with the fiber and water extracted. To arrive at 50 grams of "digestible carbohydrate," then, a person would have to eat roughly an entire bag of baby carrots! So the GI value of carrots is likely based on an entire bag. But we don't eat carrots this way. We munch on a handful or two as a snack or shred some into a salad. When it comes to assessing high-water, high-fiber foods like carrots, the portions used are much bigger than one would typically consume. This is why green veggies, which are very high in water and fiber, don't even have GI values! The testers would literally have had to have eaten several bags of them to finally consume the required "50 grams of digestible carbohydrate," so it just wasn't done.

Now close your eyes and think of various foods that we consume excessively that have virtually no water, fiber, protein, or fat. For me, sliced white bread, sugar cereals, fat-free candy, and cookies came to mind. For these foods, the GI is bang on because, unlike the peeling and dehydrating we have to do to arrive at the correct GI of an apple, we can just eat these foods as they are, no subtracting necessary!

To summarize, then, the first flaw with the GI has to do with the equivalency system (i.e., arriving at the 50-gram "digestible carbohydrate" component). Dry refined foods that are low in fiber and water have GI values that make sense, and for these types of food, the GI is an excellent and important tool. However, foods that are high in fiber and water, such as fruits and veggies, often have GI values that are falsely higher than they should be.

Let's have a look at flaw number two. When measuring the GI, we are measuring how similar the test food is to pure glucose in terms of raising blood sugar levels. If a food raises blood sugar levels quickly, it is given a high GI and is considered to be bad for us. If a food raises blood sugar levels slowly, it is given a lower GI and is considered to be better for us. But does this make sense?

Recall that fat slows the rate at which sugar is digested into our bloodstream. Fatty foods sit in our stomachs for a long time before being digested, which is why they are filling. If carbohydrates are mixed with fat, then it is harder for the digestive enzymes to get at the carbohydrate, and the sugars are therefore absorbed more slowly. Thus, the more fat a carbohydrate food contains, the lower its GI. So a piece of heavily buttered toast (i.e., fat mixed with carbohydrate) will have a lower GI than a piece of plain toast without the added fat! Read this again. Surely this does not mean that buttered toast is better for us than plain toast, or does it?

Let's look at another example, potato chips. Potato chips have a lower GI than watermelon! We all know that fat-laden potato chips are not healthier than watermelon, so why the lower GI? Because watermelon is high in water and low in fat. The qualities that render this fruit a healthy choice intuitively are the same qualities that give it a high, and therefore unhealthy, GI rating. Long story short: the GI system is flawed.

Years of research and personal experiences have shown us that high-fat diets are linked to weight gain, diabetes, heart disease, and cancers. You just don't see athletes walking around devouring potato chips and swearing off fruits and veggies, now, do you?

GI values also don't differentiate between different types of fat! For instance, which is better, olive oil or butter? GI values won't tell us. As you can see, eating solely based on the GI value of foods is not a good approach to weight loss and health promotion.

Finally, and most importantly, the GI system does not reflect how people eat normally. We don't eat portion sizes of carbohydrate foods based on the fiber, fat, protein, and water being factored out. Further, we don't eat foods in isolation. As soon as we combine one food with another, as we do when we eat meals, the GI values are no longer accurate as the ratio of fats, proteins, and carbohydrates become altered.

Now that we have reviewed the popular diets, we can appreciate the factor that links the merits of all of them. WATER! Further, we can see that when diets fail to appreciate the water content of food, they don't work. The Hershberg Diet, with its emphasis on this vital "fourth macronutrient" and "hotty" properties, will help get us back on track.

PART TWO

THE HERSHBERG DIET WEIGHT-LOSS PLAN

CHAPTER 4

LET'S REVIEW

Congratulations! You have made it to Part Two. You'll now learn how the three concepts taught in Part One can be combined to create an easy, delicious, and sustainable weight-loss plan. First, let's quickly review these three concepts:

1. **The "Fourth Macronutrient"** Water is the "fourth macronutrient." It is a critical, often-forgotten component of food, yet must be considered for weight loss. The more water a food contains, the better it is for weight loss. This concept was explained in Chapter 1.

2. **The "Hotty" Effect** "Hotty" foods are excellent for weight loss because eating these foods encourages the body to heat up and burn calories. Incorporating "hotty" foods into our diets will help us lose weight. Some "hotty" foods can even activate fat-melting hormones. This concept was explained in Chapter 2.

3. **The Hormonal Effect**   When overeaten or eaten improperly, foods that spike blood sugar and insulin levels can create a hormonal situation in the body that encourages the body to store fat, even when you're not eating. For optimal weight loss, you must eat a diet that encourages the body to handle insulin properly and activates hormones that promote weight loss. This concept was explained in Chapter 3.

CHAPTER 5

ALCOHOL

Before we get started, let's discuss how alcohol fits into the Hershberg Diet weight-loss plan.

Alcohol certainly isn't a dieter's best friend (think of a "beer belly"). But the Hershberg Diet is not about deprivation; it is meant to be easy to implement and sustain. You can drink alcohol on this diet plan as long as you have appropriate strategies to ensure that you do not jeopardize your weight-loss goals.

Using your knowledge of the three concepts introduced thus far, you'll know that the best foods and drinks for weight loss are those that are high in water, are "hotty," and have the right hormonal effect. How does alcohol rate?

Alcohol causes us to lose water. It inhibits the hormone that causes us to hold onto water. This is why we make so many bathroom trips when we drink alcohol! This is also why we feel hungover and dehydrated following a night of drinking. So when drinking alcohol, we must increase the water factor. Forgo mixed drinks completely, as most mixes are either concentrated sugar or fat. Or simply drink your beverage on the rocks or mixed with water. If you must have a mixed drink, choose a vegetable juice mixer like olive juice or Clamato or tomato juice. Also, consume a glass of water for every alcoholic drink consumed.

Alcohol can cause unstable blood sugar levels. In fact, it can spike and drop blood sugar levels rapidly and excessively. This is one reason why we crave so many simple high-sugar carbohydrates (chips, pretzels, pizza, etc.) when we drink! Our bodies are likely trying to quickly raise our blood sugar levels back up to normal. As you can see, when we add the calories consumed from drinking with the calories consumed from these foods, it's no surprise that weight gain often ensues! To combat this, drink alcohol slowly following a meal that contains some starchy carbohydrates such as whole wheat breads, pasta, rice, or legumes. *Do not* skip dinner or skimp on carbs before drinking; it will not save calories but will set you up for a late night high-sugar binge! The other trick that you may use when drinking is one that the stars often use, or so I've heard, to make it through a long night of drinking at an awards show or event. Swallow 1 tablespoon of olive or flaxseed oil (or take two flaxseed or fish oil supplements) before drinking. The fat will slow the rate of alcohol absorption; you will crave fewer high-sugar foods and feel less hungover the following day.

Alcohol may cause us to confuse what's "hotty" and what's not. To increase the "hotty" potential when drinking, get active. Dance! This way you will burn off some of the calories that you are consuming.

Most importantly, drink in moderation! While it is best to limit alcohol as much as possible when trying to lose weight, if you must imbibe, it is suggested that you limit your consumption.

If you follow these rules, you should be able to enjoy alcohol without compromising your weight-loss and health goals.

TIPS

⇨ Say no to all sugary and fatty mixed drinks.

⇨ Wine and light beers are good options.

⇨ Drink a glass of water for every alcoholic drink consumed.

⇨ Do not skip dinner or skimp on carbohydrates before drinking.

⇨ Consume complex carbohydrates (like the ones that will be introduced in Phase Two) before or along with alcohol or have 1 tablespoon (15 mL) of olive or flaxseed oil (or two fish oil or flaxseed oil supplements) before drinking.

⇨ Drink in moderation.

Now you are ready to embark on the the Hershberg Diet weight-loss plan. You will learn how to use the three concepts for optimal weight loss and health. This information will change the way you approach food and eating for life!

THE INITIATION PHASE

Phase One is a two-week initiation phase. It is the strictest phase of the diet and is designed to cleanse your body and jump-start weight loss. Foods high in the "fourth macronutrient" are emphasized in this phase. So in this phase your diet will consist mostly of high-water fruits, veggies, dairy products, fish, chicken, and meats. Because the foods suggested are high in water and therefore the best for weight loss, I encourage you to eat as much as you need to feel full and satisfied. There is no counting or tracking required. That said, your meals should still be of reasonable size, enough to satisfy your hunger but no more than that. You should feel comfortable following meals, not bursting or overstuffed.

Read the list of "Foods to Enjoy in Phase One" carefully. Stock your fridge, freezer, and pantry with these foods so that you always have them on hand. These foods should always make up the majority of your diet, no matter which phase you are in.

After you become familiar with the list of Phase One foods, read the information that follows on their associated health benefits and weight-loss properties.

In the following sections, you will find an extensive collection of easy-to-make and delicious recipes as well as a sample 14-day menu plan. You can follow the meal plan exactly for two weeks or simply use it for meal ideas.

By the time the phase ends, you will notice a significant change in your body; unhealthy high-sugar cravings will be reduced and your body will already begin to look and feel better as fat is lost and water retention decreases.

Contrary to intuition, eating high-water foods results in body water loss (diuresis) as opposed to body water gain (swelling). Here's an easy way to understand this principle.

Our bodies must keep the concentration of solutes, such as sodium and potassium, incredibly stable. This is done by altering the amount of solvent—body water. Think about it: if you put a tablespoon of salt in a glass of water, what's the easiest way to make it taste saltier? By pouring out some of the water—this increases the concentration of salt (sodium). Now, because water plays such an important role in regulating solute concentrations, our bodies store excess water for this purpose (in our ankles, hands, hips, bellies, etc.) just in case it's not available from our diets. So just like our bodies are designed to store fat to protect us from starvation, our bodies store water to protect us from dehydration. Now, when the majority of our diets consist of high-water foods, the body senses that it is at no threat of dehydration, so it feels confident that it can shed some of the extra water that it had been storing. The result? Eating high-water foods will help you lose excess water weight—you feel thinner, less bloated, and your blood pressure decreases.

Foods to Enjoy in Phase One

While all of the following foods qualify as acceptable for Phase One, I separated them into two columns. This is because the foods in the left column are so high in water and so good for weight loss that they deserve special attention. Make your selections from this column as often as possible to speed weight loss!

Veggies—asparagus, bok choy, broccoli, brussels sprouts, burdock, celery, collard greens, cucumber, endive, green beans, green onions, hearts of palm (canned), kale, leeks, lettuce, pickles (not sweet varieties), scallions, snow peas, spinach, vegetable broth, zucchini, all herbs	**Veggies**—artichokes, beets, red and green bell peppers, carrots, cauliflower, eggplant, fennel, mushrooms, okra, olives, onion, pumpkin, radish, rhubarb, rutabaga, salsa, squash, Swiss chard, taro root, tomato, tomato sauce (no sugar added), watercress, yellow beans
Fruits—lemon, lime, all berries, grapefruit	**Fruits**—apple, avocado, banana, cantaloupe, cherries, grapes, guava, honeydew, kiwi, kumquat, loquat, nectarine, orange, papaya, passion fruit, peach, pear, persimmon, pineapple, plum, tangerine, watermelon, unsweetened applesauce, fruit-flavored sugar-free gelatine

Animal protein—egg whites (or low-fat liquid egg substitutes); beef or chicken broth	**Animal protein**—chicken and turkey without skin (white meat); fish and seafood (those packed in oil, battered, deep fried, or mixed with butter/cream sauce don't count); lean cuts of red meat (pork, veal, beef, lamb) trimmed of fat; Canadian back bacon; turkey or chicken bacon; lean ground chicken and turkey; lean turkey, chicken, and ham deli meat; game meat
Vegetable protein—vegetable broth; miso soup	**Vegetable protein**—tofu (buy low-fat varieties); low-fat veggie-based meat substitutes, patties, and weiners; sugar-free low-fat soy and whey-based protein powders and drinks
Dairy—none	**Dairy**—reduced-fat milk and soy milk (skim is best); fat-free, artificially sweetened yogurts (not frozen varieties); fat-free or reduced-fat cottage cheese, ricotta, or feta; fat-free sour cream; fat-free, artificially sweetened frozen treats (must have less than 50 calories per bar)

Drinks— water, green tea, black tea	**Drinks**—vegetable juice, light or diet fruit-flavored juice, diet hot chocolate, coffee, diet soft drinks
Fats—fat-free or butter-flavored cooking spray	**Fats**—olive oil, flaxseed oil, canola oil, vegetable oil, sesame oil, safflower oil, sunflower oil, non-hydrogenated light margarine, reduced-fat salad dressings, reduced-fat mayonnaise

Extras Hot peppers, mustard, cinnamon, garlic, ginger, vinegars, soy sauce, sugar substitutes, any other herb or spice (including seasoning salts)

Vegetables As you may recall from our romaine lettuce example in Chapter 1, most vegetables can be considered "waters" because so much of their weight is made up of zero-calorie water! Additionally, many veggies contain fiber. We must work to digest that fiber, which burns calories. Most veggies, provided they are not cooked with fat or dipped in fatty or sugary sauces, can help us lose weight just by eating them! If that's not hot, I don't know what is! Stock your fridge, freezer, and pantry with fresh, frozen, and canned veggies and include them at meals and snacks as often as possible.

TIPS

➪ Eat veggies raw, steamed, or boiled to preserve water content.

➪ Consume salads with meals as a side dish rather than before the meal. You will eat much less this way and your meal will be more satisfying.

➪ The veggies in the left column of the preceding chart are especially high in water. When you eat them, you may even burn more calories than you consume! Include these at meals as often as possible to maximize weight loss.

➪ Asparagus, cucumber, and parsley are excellent natural mild diuretics that can help us shed water weight.

➪ Pickles are virtually calorie-free, although they do contain a lot of salt. Too much salt can make you bloat, so be careful!

➪ Olives are higher in fat and salt than most other veggies, but they are extremely nutritious. Unless you eat them in excessive quantities, olives (less than five per serving) can be part of any smart weight-loss plan!

➪ My new favorite veggie is spaghetti squash. It is the perfect substitute for pasta, hence its name! I make dishes like squash pizza (I use a layer of baked squash instead of dough). I make a delicious squash lasagna— and even squash pie! Read the following recipe section to learn how to use this wonder veggie. Although it is slightly more caloric than some other veggies, it is more filling and therefore the perfect replacement for low-water, low-"hotty," and insulin-spiking starches like white bread, pasta, and rice.

⇨ We know that tomatoes are high in water and excellent for weight loss. However, a substance in tomatoes called lycopene has also been shown to help fight prostate cancer, the most common cancer in men.

⇨ Be careful when consuming canned vegetable soups and sauces, as many of them contain plenty of added sugar and salt. Check the ingredient list or nutrition label to ensure that sugar isn't on the list, or simply make your own.

Fruits If you are among the many people who avoided fruits, erroneously thinking that they were too high in sugar to facilitate weight loss, get ready to enjoy these sweet natural delicacies again. Fruits are among the highest-water, -fiber, and "-hotty" foods around—so they can help us lose weight! You will be amazed at how good you start to feel when you incorporate fruit into your diet. Even better, your craving for high-sugar junk foods will drastically diminish as you incorporate fruit into your diet. Because fruit can be higher in sugar than the other Phase One foods, I suggest you have **no more than 2 per day** when choosing from the right column.

While whole fruits help with weight loss, fruit juices do not! Juices are higher in sugar because many fruits have to be sqeezed to get the juice–when we eat the fruit, we eat the juice plus the high-fiber peel, rind, and seeds. The juice lacks the fiber and "hotty" properties of the fruits from which they are made. When we take the fiber out, we speed the absorption of sugar into our blood. Eat the fruit; ditch the juice!

Dried fruits are low-water. (They are dried!) They are therefore very concentrated forms of sugar and calories and should be avoided. Sorry, but no raisins, dried cranberries, or any other dried fruit that you can think of allowed in Phase One.

TIPS

⇨ Lemons and limes are acidic citrus fruits. Acid helps slow the absorption of sugar into the blood and thus helps to create the proper hormonal effect. Also, these foods are so high in water that they can be considered calorie-free! Squeeze lemons and limes into water and tea and over foods to maximize weight loss.

⇨ Berries contain a lot of water and insoluble (indigestible) fiber. They are therefore among the lowest-calorie foods. Berries must be eaten fresh or frozen and never dried or with added sugar.

⇨ As you may recall from Chapter 1, grapefruit is essentially a water with fiber. Sweeten it with a sugar substitute such as Splenda or stevia mixed with cinnamon to maintain the "hotty" effect.

⇨ Avocados are higher in fat than other fruits. However, they are excellent sources of vitamin C, folic acid, and potassium. So while I encourage you to eat this delectable fruit, do so infrequently, and in smaller quantities than the other fruits.

⇨ Bananas are somewhat drier and therefore can be higher in calories than other fruits. However, they are very good sources of potassium, an electrolyte that is critical for our bodies. Try to eat bananas somewhat less often than other fruits.

Protein The proteins listed earlier are high-water by virtue of their chemical structure and low fat content. They are also "hotty" as they are complex and require a lot of work in the body to break them down. Further, they do not cause spikes in blood sugar or insulin, so they help to create the proper hormonal effect. Notice that I have not included dried beans and lentils as protein sources appropriate for Phase One. While these are excellent sources of plant-based protein with disease-fighting and "hotty" properties, they will be introduced in Phase Two, because they can be concentrated sources of calories when overeaten. If you are a vegetarian or vegan, however, you may consider lentils and dried beans as Phase One foods to ensure that you are receiving adequate protein.

TIPS

⇨ When choosing cuts of meat, look for the words "round" or "loin" in the name. These varieties, such as striploin, sirloin, tenderloin, and eye of round, are usually the lowest in "water-hating" fat. Fat repels water—i.e., oil and water don't mix, so foods high in fat are often lower in water! Or simply ask the butcher for the lowest-fat cuts. Always trim and discard any visible fat and use low-fat cooking techniques, spices and seasonings that are flavorful yet fat-free, and healthy oils (see right column of the preceding chart).

⇨ Lean sources of red meat are very rich sources of easily absorbable iron. Diets low in iron can lead to low blood levels and feelings of fatigue and low energy.

⇨ Give grass-fed, as opposed to grain-fed, cuts of meat a try. Imagine a high-water food eating a high-water food . . . wow!

⇨ Many people are concerned that seafood such as prawns and squid raises blood cholesterol levels. However, these foods are extremely high in omega-3 fatty acids and low in saturated fat. Omega-3 fatty acids have been shown to decrease the risk of heart attack, stroke, and inflammation. The cholesterol contained in seafood is therefore offset by their high-water, low-saturated-fat content and disease-fighting properties. In fact, omega-3 fatty acids are so good for us that many cardiologists now recommend taking fish oil supplements!

⇨ When preparing poultry, meat, and fish, use modest amounts of healthy fats like olive oil or cooking spray. Use tomato-based sauces instead of cream or butter sauces. Use herbs and spices to enhance flavor. Use low-fat, water-preserving cooking techniques such as poaching, boiling, steaming, and microwaving as often as possible.

Dairy The dairy products listed in the preceding chart contain an excellent healthy combination of protein and carbohydrate. The protein helps slow the absorption of milk sugar into our blood, which helps stabilize insulin levels, thus creating a good hormonal effect. The protein also helps to keep "hotty" potential high. The low-fat nature of these products ensures that the "water-hating" fat has been removed, making them less caloric and much better for weight loss.

TIPS

⇨ Dairy products contain calcium, which we need to keep our bones strong and healthy. Osteoporosis (thin, weak bones) affects many individuals at some point in their lives and has a high associated mortality rate, so getting calcium in our diet is very important.

⇨ Studies show that diets high in low-fat dairy products are associated with both weight and fat loss.

⇨ Including fat-free yogurt and milk in our diet (or calcium supplements) can help us beat the bloat. Calcium is exchanged for sodium (salt) in our bodies. So the more calcium we consume, the more salt we should shed. When we shed salt, water goes along with it and, voila, we're beating the bloat! This is a great trick for premenstrual bloating and has even been shown to decrease menstrual cramps as well!

Drinks   The drinks listed above are extremely high in water. However, that does not mean that they are all created equal.

TIPS

⇨ When we drink ice-cold water, our bodies must do work to warm the water to body temperature. This requires that the body produces heat ("hotty")! Thus, we actually burn calories when we drink cold water.

⇨ **Note:** While drinking beverages cold may help you burn a few additional calories, please note that if you have digestive troubles, you may want to avoid this, as according to traditional modalities of eating (Indian and Chinese), drinking beverages at room temperature is preferable for digestion.

⇨ Studies have shown that drinking green tea will cause our bodies to burn calories as heat ("hotty"), activate our fat-burning hormones, and slow the absorption of sugar into the blood. Drink green tea often to expedite weight loss.

⇨ Green tea inhibits amylase, the enzyme that breaks down carbohydrates, so it can reduce the amount of carbohydrate digested. This allows us to dispose of some of the carbohydrate calories we've ingested! Green tea is also great for curbing cravings for sweets. Try it. The next time you crave a sweet, have a glass of green tea first and see what happens!

⇨ If you add sugar and fat to coffee and tea, you add calories. I used to waste calories by mindlessly adding cream and sugar to my morning coffee. Now I simply add skim milk. You'll be amazed at how quickly your palate adapts. The thought of sugar in my coffee now makes me cringe. If you want to jazz up your java, use flavor enhancers like cinnamon, nutmeg, vanilla extract, and artificial sweetener.

⇨ Many people confuse the sensations of hunger and thirst. Have you ever eaten platefuls of Chinese food, only to feel hungry an hour or two later? Chinese food can be extremely high in sodium (salt), which is dehydrating. Our bodies may actually be thirsty for water rather than hungry for more food; we just mistake the sensations, which leads us to overconsume. The next time you feel hungry, have a glass of water first and re-evaluate. Remember, if you drink the water-ice cold, you'll actually burn calories while wondering whether or not you're hungry!

Fats Although I have included fats in Phase One, this category must be approached differently than the others. This is because fat, by virtue of its chemical structure, repels water (oil and water don't mix). However, not all fats are created equal. Monosaturated and polyunsaturated fats, like the ones often found in high-water foods such as fish and vegetables, are very good for our health and have therefore been selected as appropriate for Phase One. While they should not be consumed in excessive quantities, when used in moderation they can help promote weight loss by helping keep us full and slowing the absorption of sugar into our blood. So fats help the body stabilize blood sugar and insulin levels, thus creating a positive hormonal environment. Use the fats listed above to cook and dress foods, but use them sparingly (try for no more than 3 tablespoons per day). Use fat-free cooking sprays and nonstick cookware whenever possible to reduce the amount of added fat.

Reduced-fat salad dressings and mayonnaises have also been included in this category. Although they are labeled as lower in fat, many of them still contain quite a bit. Moreover, most contain quite a lot of sugar. So when using these dressings, watch your serving size. I recommend not using more than 2–3 tablespoons of salad dressing per salad. I mix 2 tablespoons of low-fat salad dressing with an equal part of vinegar and then dress my salads. Similarly, I often mix

1 tablespoon low-fat mayonnaise with some vinegar when mixing tuna salad. I find this dilution trick quite helpful, as I have been known to consume giant salads, which obviously need more than 2–3 tablespoons of dressing! Use your own judgment, as there are a wide variety of salad dressings available. I will list a few of my favorites later in the book. Stick to dressings that have less than 30 calories per tablespoon. Of course, when you have time, it is always best to make your own fresh dressings using ingredients such as the healthy oils listed earlier plus vinegars, herbs, and even berries and a sugar substitute if necessary.

TIPS

⇨ Cooking and butter-flavored sprays are low enough in calories that you needn't worry about quantity. For the rest of the listed fats, try not to exceed 3 tablespoons per day. Although these are healthy fats that our bodies need, they still contain 9 calories per gram, roughly 120 calories per tablespoon

⇨ Use chicken, veggie or beef stock or fat-free Italian dressing to "sauté" foods wherever possible

⇨ Substitute the healthy fats listed above for less healthy fats such as butter wherever possible.

Extras In addition to being virtually calorie-free, many of the "extras" permitted in Phase One can actually help increase weight loss through their "hotty" properties! Use these "extras" as freely as you like and jump-start weight loss.

TIPS

➡ It should come as no surprise that hot peppers, such as chili peppers and cayenne pepper, and hot mustard are "hotty!" In fact, these foods are such "hotties" that we feel hot after eating them! If you can handle the spice, go for it. You will burn extra calories when consuming these items.

➡ Eating ginger can raise our metabolism and help us burn off calories as heat because ginger causes our body temperature to increase. It's "hotty" indeed! Use fresh ginger in stir-fries, with fish, or in a tea.

➡ Cinnamon is my favorite spice and a dieter's best friend. I mix cinnamon with Splenda or stevia and sprinkle it on oatmeal, fruit and my morning coffee. It's even great on tomato sauce, squash, and sweet potatoes. (Note: oatmeal and sweet potatoes will be introduced in Phase Two).

➡ Soy sauce has a lot of salt, which can cause bloating. Opt for low-sodium varieties whenever possible.

➡ Stock up on different flavors of vinegars, such as red wine, white wine, apple cider, balsamic, rice wine, and fruit. Because vinegar is high in acid and virtually calorie-free, it aids in weight loss! I combine different vinegars with a touch of olive oil, herbs, cinnamon, and Splenda to make delicious, low-calorie salad dressings.

➡ Although sugar substitutes are great calorie savers, many people worry that they are harmful. However, here is some information that may ease your mind. Aspartame, a commonly used sugar substitute, is made from protein and is 200 times sweeter than sugar, so a little goes a long way. The Canadian government has set the acceptable daily intake (ADI—the amount that is considered safe and will not cause harm) as 40 milligrams per kilogram of body weight per day. For the average person, this amounts to about 15 diet pops or 181 packets of Equal per day! Sucralose, better known as Splenda, is another common sugar substitute and is made from sugar, making it more palatable and better suited for baking. The ADI for Splenda is 9 mg/kg/day. For the average person, this is roughly equivalent to 58 packets of Splenda per day!

Basic Grocery List To Get You Started

The following is a good grocery list to get you started; read the Phase One ingredients and recipes and pick up any additional ingredients that you need.

Dairy:
Skim milk
Artificially sweetened, fat-free yogurt and mousses—assorted flavors (Danone and Silhouette make great-tasting yogurts)
Reduced-fat feta cheese
Fat-free cottage cheese
Fat-free sour cream
Reduced-fat ricotta cheese

Condiments, herbs and spices, and dressings and oils:
Cinnamon
Splenda (artificial sugar substitute)
Brown sugar substitute (e.g., Sugar Twin)
Soy sauce
Sesame oil
Olive oil
Cooking spray
I Can't Believe It's Not Butter! Spray or Becel Topping and Cooking Spray
Balsamic vinegar
Rice wine vinegar
White wine vinegar
Fat-free mayonnaise

Reduced-fat salad dressings (eg. Newman's Own Low Fat Sesame
Thai Dressing, Renee's Poppy Seed Light and Renee's Caesar Light
Dressings are excellent)
Dill
Parsley
Cayenne powder
Ginger—fresh or frozen
Garlic
Olives
Lemon juice

Vegetables
Iceberg lettuce
Romaine lettuce
Mixed bags of assorted lettuces
Cabbage
Red onion
Tomatoes—whole, grape, and/or cherry tomatoes
Celery
Carrots—bags of baby carrots are good to have
Green onions
Green beans
Cucumber
Asparagus (fresh and canned)
Hearts of palm (canned—expensive but delicious!)
Spaghetti squash
Broccoli
Cauliflower
Mushrooms (assorted varieties)
Frozen spinach
Frozen bags of mixed vegetables (great for stir-fries)

Fruits
Fresh and/or frozen berries (eg. blueberries, blackberries, raspber-
ries, and strawberries)
Apples
Oranges
Grapefruit
Pears
Grapes

Protein
Skinless, boneless chicken breasts
Lean ground chicken and turkey
Assorted fish (eg. tilapia, salmon, halibut, cod)
Low-fat firm tofu
Fat-free or low-fat deli meats (e.g., turkey, ham, chicken)
Soy and whey-based protein powder (choose one that is low-fat and
artificially sweetened)
Low-fat precooked bacon (chicken or ham bacon—Piller's Maple
Flavor Smoked Ham has only 1 gram of fat per serving and tastes
great)
Canned tuna, packed in water

Soups
Vegetable broth
Miso soup, packaged
Chicken and beef broth

Desserts
Diet gelatin (e.g., diet Jell-O)
Reduced-fat, artificially sweetened frozen treats (fat-free
Creamsicles and Fudgsicles are great if they have less than 50 calo-
ries per bar.)
Diet or light hot chocolate

Beverages

Water

Green tea

Sparkling water (e.g., Perrier)

Diet soda

Diet flavor crystals (e.g., Crystal Lite)

Coffee

PHASE ONE

APPROPRIATE RECIPES

Now that you know which foods are suitable for Phase One, let's look at some recipe ideas appropriate for this phase. Some of these recipes will be included in the 14-day sample menu plan to follow.

BREAKFAST

∝ Basic Egg White Omelette

Remember, egg whites are very high in water and easy to prepare, so definitely include them when trying to lose weight.

4 to 5	egg whites or 4 to 5 oz (120 to 150 g) low-fat liquid egg substitute (I buy mine in the carton so I don't have to fuss with cracking eggs and discarding yolks) Cooking spray Salt and freshly ground black pepper 9-inch (23 cm) microwave-safe dish with a cover	4 to 5

Spray dish with cooking spray. Pour in as much egg white as you want. Sprinkle with salt and pepper. Cover. Microwave on high for about 3 minutes (cooking times may vary depending on your microwave's power).

A perfect omelette—better and easier to clean up than one made in a frying pan! This method is a real time-saver in the morning, as you can dress and get organized while your breakfast is cooking.

If you want to add cheese, cook the eggs as above. Remove cover, add cheese (use feta in Phase One; other low-fat cheeses will be introduced in Phase Two), cover and let sit for a minute or so until cheese melts.

This is the basic recipe; you can add other ingredients to the egg whites before microwaving. Experiment with different veggies, putting them in the covered dish with the egg whites—the veggies will steam as the omelette cooks. Here are some of my favorites to help you get started.

Options

Asparagus, Feta, and Olives Chop fresh asparagus stems and tips, discarding the woody bottoms. Add to the egg whites, cover and microwave. Remove lid, add feta cheese and sliced olives, cover and let sit for a minute to melt the cheese and heat the olives. Enjoy!

Bacon and Green Onion Cut low-fat precooked bacon (or low-fat chicken or ham bacon) into small pieces. Slice green onion. Add both to egg whites, then microwave for 3 minutes. Perfecto!

Herbs Add fresh herbs like parsley, dill, or basil to the egg whites before microwaving for 3 minutes. Tasty, filling, and very healthy.

❧ Basic Smoothie

This is another delicious and easy-to-make breakfast staple.

1	container (6 oz/170 g) sugar-free fat-free yogurt, any flavor	1
⅓ cup	cold water	75 mL
⅓ cup	fresh or frozen berries	75 mL
⅓ cup	low-fat firm tofu	75 mL
1 tbsp	Splenda Cinnamon to taste	15 mL

Place yogurt, water, berries and tofu in blender. Add Splenda, some sprinkles of cinnamon and blend to desired texture. Add ice if you like.

Don't worry if you don't love tofu. It thickens the smoothie, adds protein, and simply takes on the flavor of the fruit and yogurt. Tofu can also be replaced by banana, if desired.

❧ Basic Protein Shake

1 cup	fresh or frozen berries	250 mL
2 tbsp	sugar-free protein powder	30 mL
1 cup	cold water	250 mL
1 tbsp	flaxseed oil (optional)	15 mL
	Sugar substitute (stevia or Splenda) to taste	

Place berries, protein powder, water, oil, and sugar substitute in blender and blend until creamy. Add ice and enjoy!

LUNCH AND DINNER

SALADS

Salads can be mixed to taste—add more of one ingredient that you like and less of another that you don't.

✍ Basic Tuna Salad

	White wine vinegar	
	Fat-free mayonnaise	
1	can (6 oz/170 g) tuna packed in water, drained	1
	Green onions, chopped	
	Celery, chopped	
	Salt and freshly ground black pepper	

Add vinegar to mayo and then combine mayonnaise mixture, tuna, green onions, celery, and salt and pepper. Serve with a squeeze of lemon, if you like.

✍ Iceberg Lettuce Wrap

1	head iceberg lettuce	1

Discard any damaged or discolored outer leaves. Cut lettuce in half. Carefully peel off outer leaves. Use three layers of leaves per wrap so that it is strong enough to hold a filling. This is an excellent substitute for bread.

&. Greek Salad

Delicious topped with grilled chicken, deli chicken or turkey, or even canned tuna.

> Iceberg lettuce, chopped
> Red onion, sliced
> Tomatoes, sliced
> Olives, black or Kalamata
> Green bell pepper, sliced
> Light feta cheese, crumbled

Combine lettuce, red onion, tomatoes, olives, bell pepper and feta in a bowl.

DRESSING

Use Basic Balsamic Dressing (see recipe, page 103) or any low-fat Greek dressing (diluted with balsamic vinegar).

Note: Greek salad can be an excellent choice at a restaurant, provided that you ask for the dressing on the side. Because restaurants tend to use a lot of feta, which adds taste and texture, I find that balsamic vinegar is all that is needed to dress the salad.

⁊ஐ Cobb Salad

Romaine lettuce, chopped
Iceberg lettuce, chopped
Cooked or deli-style chicken or turkey
Hard-cooked egg white
Turkey or chicken bacon, cooked and crumbled
Whole tomatoes, chopped, or cherry tomatoes, halved
Avocado, peeled and sliced (remember, avocados
are high in fat compared to other fruits, so don't
overdo it)

Combine lettuces, chicken, egg white, bacon, tomatoes, and avocado in a bowl.

DRESSING
Use Sweet Balsamic Dressing or Tangy Mustard Dressing, (see recipes, pages 103 and 105). Store-bought low-fat honey mustard dressing also works well. Remember to dilute the dressing with a vinegar of your choice.

ᐊ Warm Asian Chicken Salad

DRESSING

2 tbsp	sesame oil	30 mL
2 tbsp	rice wine vinegar	30 mL
2 tbsp	low-sodium soy sauce	30 mL
2 tbsp	Splenda	30 mL

SALAD

Skinless, boneless chicken breasts, sliced

Water chestnuts (these are very high in water, are great in salads, and add tons of crunch)

Iceberg lettuce, chopped

Baby spinach

Bean sprouts

Snow peas

Cucumber, sliced

DRESSING

To make dressing, combine the sesame oil, rice wine vinegar, soy sauce, and Splenda in a small bowl and set aside.

SALAD

Heat frying pan and spray with cooking spray. Add chicken to pan and sauté. When brown, add in the dressing and the water chestnuts. Continue to sauté until chicken and water chestnuts are done. Meanwhile, toss lettuce, spinach, bean sprouts, snow peas, and cucumber to make a salad. Pour cooked chicken mixture over salad and enjoy!

✒ Asian-Style Cucumber

1	English cucumber, peeled and sliced	1
1 tbsp	rice wine vinegar	15 mL
2 tsp	soy sauce	10 mL
1 tsp	sesame oil	5 mL
	Sugar substitute to taste	

Combine cucumber, vinegar, soy sauce, and sesame oil in a small bowl. Add sugar substitute to taste.

✒ Coleslaw

1	red cabbage, quartered and thinly sliced	1
1	red onion, thinly sliced	1
⅓ cup	fat-free sour cream	75 mL
⅓ cup	fat-free mayonnaise	75 mL
1 tbsp	balsamic vinegar	15 mL
1 tbsp	white wine vinegar	15 mL
1 tsp	dried tarragon	5 mL
	Sugar substitute to taste	
	salt and freshly ground black pepper to taste	

Mix cabbage, red onion, sour cream, mayonnaise, vinegars, tarragon, sugar substitute, and salt and pepper in a large bowl. Refrigerate for at least 6 hours to allow flavors to blend.

❧ Grilled Portobello Mushrooms

	Balsamic vinegar	
	Fat-free Italian dressing	
	Salt and freshly ground black pepper	
	Basil	
4–5	Portobello mushrooms	4–5

Whisk together vinegar, Italian dressing, salt, pepper, and basil. Pour over portobellos.

Line a cookie sheet with foil and spray with cooking spray. Place mushrooms on sheet and bake for approximately 20 minutes.

SALAD DRESSINGS

❧ Basic Balsamic Dressing

Makes about 1 cup (250 mL) of dressing (to make 1 serving, quarter the recipe).

¼ cup	olive oil	60 mL
¼ cup	balsamic vinegar	60 mL
1–2	cloves garlic, minced	1–2
	Salt and freshly ground black pepper to taste	
	Fresh or dried basil to taste	

Place oil, vinegar, garlic, salt, pepper, and basil in a jar with lid, shake well, and refrigerate. Alternatively, you can place in a blender and add berries and Splenda for a delicious sweet version.

❧ Sweet Balsamic Dressing

Makes about 1 cup (250 mL) of dressing (to make 1 serving, quarter the recipe)

¼ cup	olive oil	60 mL
¼ cup	balsamic vinegar (or raspberry vinegar)	60 mL
¼ cup	water	60 mL
¼ cup	Splenda	60 mL
¼ cup	fat-free sugar-free plain yogurt	60 mL
Pinch	salt and freshly ground black pepper	Pinch

Place oil, vinegar, water, Splenda, yogurt, salt, and pepper in a jar with lid. Shake well and refrigerate.

🙠 Oriental Dressing

This is also a great sauce to sauté veggies, chicken, and beef.
Makes 1 cup.

1 tbsp	reduced-sodium soy sauce	15 mL
1 tbsp	sesame oil	15 mL
⅓ cup	rice wine vinegar	75 mL
2 tbsp	grated fresh ginger	30 mL
1	clove garlic, minced	1
1 tsp	cornstarch	5 mL
	Sugar substitute (Splenda or stevia) to taste	

Bring soy sauce, sesame oil, vinegar, ginger, garlic, cornstarch, and sugar substitute to a boil in a saucepan over medium-high heat. Cook for about 1 minute, until slightly thickened. Cool to room temperature.

⋙ Tangy Mustard Dressing

¼ cup	white wine vinegar	60 mL
3 tbsp	Splenda	45 mL
1 tsp	olive oil	5 mL
1 tsp	Dijon mustard	5 mL
2 tbsp	fat-free sugar-free plain yogurt	30 mL

Whisk together vinegar, Splenda, oil, mustard, and yogurt in a small bowl.

⋙ Sesame Dressing

2 tbsp	chicken broth	30 mL
1½ tbsp	rice or white wine vinegar	22 mL
1½ tbsp	soy sauce	22 mL
1 tbsp	sesame oil	15 mL
	Splenda to taste	

Whisk together broth, vinegar, soy sauce, sesame oil, and Splenda in a small bowl.

SOUPS

Breakthrough Mushroom Soup

This recipe is fantastic! It makes a large pot of soup that is delicious, filling, and so good for you. You can freeze portions for when you don't feel like cooking.

3	packages (½ oz/15 g each) dried mushrooms	3
2 tbsp	olive oil	30 mL
	Cooking spray	
1	onion	1
4 cups	chicken stock	1 L
1½ lbs	fresh mushrooms, sliced (shiitakes taste best, but regular button mushrooms can be used to reduce cost)	700 g
¼ cup	skim (2% if you like it a little creamier) milk	60 mL
¼ cup	dry sherry	60 mL
	Salt and freshly ground black pepper to taste	

Boil 3 cups (750 mL) of water and remove from heat. Soak dried mushrooms in the hot water for 30 minutes.

Meanwhile, in a large saucepan, heat olive oil and sauté chopped onion for 5–7 minutes, until golden. Add fresh mushrooms and cook for 3 minutes.

Strain the soaked mushrooms over a bowl and reserve the liguid. Add 2 cups (500 mL) of this drained liquid along with the chicken stock to the saucepan. Stir in the drained mushrooms. Simmer for 20 minutes. Remove from heat.

Transfer the mixture to a blender or food processor and purée in batches. Add the puréed soup back into the saucepan. Add ¼ the milk, ¼ sherry, and salt and pepper to taste. Cook for another 3 minutes.

You can eat the soup right away or freeze for later use. Enjoy. You will love this recipe!

℞ The Best Homemade Chicken Soup

This takes some time to make, but it's worth it! You'll have tons to refrigerate and freeze for later use. Great for a quick, healthy meal!

1	chicken, at least 3–4 lbs, cut up into 8 or 9 pieces	1
1 tbsp	salt, or more to taste	15 mL
	freshly ground black pepper	
1	bunch fresh parsley	1
1	bunch fresh dill	1
1	bunch celery	1
1½–2 lbs	carrots (about 8 to 12 medium)	700 to 900 g
1½–2 lbs	onions (about 4 to 6 medium)	700 to 900 g
2–3	parsnips (skip these in Phase One but add them in Phase Two)	2–3
	Salt and freshly ground pepper	

Put chicken in the bottom of a large pot, cover with water and add salt. The pot should be less than two-thirds full. Bring to a full boil over high heat. Skim off any foam and discard.

Add the pepper, parsley, dill, and celery heart, leaves, and a few stalks.

Cut one-quarter of the carrots and onions (and 1 parsnip, if using) into chunks. Add to the pot.

Simmer for 3 hours, adding water as necessary to keep the pot two-thirds full. If you have a fat skimmer, repeatedly skim off the fat that comes to the top.

Remove from heat; strain out chicken and vegetables. If you didn't skim off the fat, you'll have to leave the soup in the refrigerator to chill (probably overnight), until the fat on top solidifies. It can then be lifted off easily.

Dice remaining celery, carrots, and parsnips (if using).

Return soup to a boil, add chopped vegetables and simmer for about ½ hour more. Meanwhile, remove chicken from bones, chop the meat and return to soup. (The vegetables used in making the stock can be eaten as is or chopped and added back to soup.)

Add salt and pepper to taste.

FISH AND MEAT ENTRÉES

Basic Fish

Spray microwave-safe dish with cooking spray and lay fish (cod, tilapia, halibut, sole, or salmon, frozen or fresh) on bottom. Sprinkle fish with salt, pepper, fresh or dried (either-or, although fresh is always better) dill, and freshly squeezed lemon. Cover dish with plastic wrap, leaving a corner open for steam to escape. Microwave on high for 3–5 minutes, until fish flakes. That's it! Nothing could be easier. I find that fish cooks best in the microwave—and it's so quick and easy to do. Experiment with different sauces, marinades, and spices to add flavor. You can also add veggies—such as broccoli, onions, peppers, asparagus, cucumbers, etc., to the fish before microwaving. They steam perfectly and infuse the fish with flavors. An entire meal in just a few minutes!

Tilapia Pockets

Makes 4 servings.

2 tbsp	balsamic vinegar	30 mL
¼ cup	Newman's Own Light Thai Sesame Dressing (or another light marinade)	60 mL
4	tilapia fillets, cut into ½-inch (1 cm) strips	4
1	can water chestnuts, drained	1
1	bunch asparagus, woody ends trimmed	1
1	onion, sliced	1
1	green bell pepper, sliced	1
	Salt and freshly ground black pepper	

Mix the vinegar and Thai Sesame Dressing. Marinate the fish and veggies in the mixture for about 30 minutes.

Preheat the oven to 450°F (230°C).

Tear aluminum foil into 8- × 12-inch (20 × 30 cm) squares. Spray the squares with cooking spray. Arrange fish, water chestnuts, asparagus, onion, and green peppers in center of foil. Season with salt and pepper to taste. Fold sides to form a sealed packet. Place in oven directly on rack and bake for 15–25 minutes, depending on desired crunch of vegetables.

* You can use any type of fish you like; cod, halibut, and salmon would all work. Just experiment. If you don't like fish, you can use skinless, boneless chicken breast, halved and cut into ½-inch (1 cm) strips instead.

&. Tangy Tilapia
Makes 4 servings.

1 tbsp	olive oil	15 mL
1	small onion, diced	1
3	cloves garlic, minced	3
1	can 28 oz (828 mL) crushed tomatoes with juice	1
½ cup	dry white wine	125 mL
	Salt and freshly ground black pepper to taste	
	fresh or dried oregano to taste	
	fresh or dried basil to taste	
4	tilapia fillets cut into bite-size pieces (add scallops, shrimp, and/or substitute other white fish as you like)	4
4 tbsp	light feta cheese	60 mL

Heat oil in frying pan over medium heat. Sauté onion for a few minutes, until softened, then add garlic and cook for about another 1 minute. Add tomatoes, wine, salt, pepper, oregano, and basil and cook for 8–10 minutes longer, until the sauce starts to thicken. Add additional herbs to taste. Add tilapia and cook for about 4 minutes. Sprinkle with feta and serve.

⁓ Poached Salmon

Makes 2 servings.

1	bunch romaine lettuce	1
2	salmon fillets 4–6 oz each (113–170 g), skin removed	2
	Salt and freshly ground black pepper	
1 tbsp	fresh dill (or 1 tsp/5 mL dried)	15 mL
1 tbsp	freshly squeezed lemon juice	15 mL

Wash and dry lettuce and arrange half the leaves on bottom of microwave-safe rectangular dish. Place salmon on top. Season with salt, pepper, dill, and lemon juice. Cover with another layer of lettuce leaves. Microwave for approximately 5 minutes—salmon will flake when ready.

ᴥ Ginger Salmon

Makes 2 servings.

3 tbsp	low-sodium soy sauce	45 mL
2 tsp	sesame oil	10 mL
1 tbsp	Splenda	15 mL
¼ cup	dry sherry	60 mL
3	green onions, finely chopped	3
1 tsp	freshly grated ginger	5 mL
2	cloves garlic, minced	2
2	salmon fillets (4–6 oz each /113–170 g)	2

Combine soy sauce, sesame oil, Splenda, sherry, green onions, ginger, and garlic in a small bowl.

Spray microwave-safe dish with cooking spray. Place salmon in dish and pour marinade over. Partially cover so that steam can vent. Microwave on high for about 5 minutes, until salmon flakes. Do not eat salmon skin because it contains too much fat (BUT IT'S A GOOD FAT!).

✍ Tuna Steaks

Makes 2 servings.

2–4 tbsp	balsamic vinegar	30–60 mL
2–4 tbsp	olive oil	30–60 mL
2	tuna steaks	2
	Steak seasoning	
6	fresh rosemary sprigs, chopped	6

Preheat oven to 400°F (200°C).

Whisk balsamic vinegar and olive oil together.

Place tuna steaks in an ovenproof dish and pour marinade over. Sprinkle with steak seasoning (or salt and pepper) and rosemary.

Cook at for 3–6 minutes per side.

✍ Tofu Delight

Use as much or as little tofu as you like, depending on how much you want to make up for your fridge.

Press a block of extra-firm tofu between paper towels to absorb some of the moisture. Cut into 1-inch (2.5 cm) cubes. Place tofu cubes in a plastic container and pour in Sesame Dressing (see recipe, page 105) to taste. Refrigerate and eat cold as a snack, or sauté cubes in a frying pan, using cooking spray. Tofu Delight is also excellent to top salads or in stir-fries.

❧ "Hotty" Pork Tenderloin

1–2 lbs	pork tenderloin	450 g to 900 g
2 tbsp	sesame oil	30 mL
3 tbsp	Splenda	45 mL
2 tbsp	soy sauce	30 mL
2 cups	chicken broth	500 mL
3 tbsp	grated fresh ginger	45 mL
3	cloves garlic, minced	3

Place pork, sesame oil, Splenda, soy sauce, chicken broth, ginger, and garlic in a large bowl and marinate for at least a few hours, but preferably overnight. Drain and discard marinade.

Preheat oven to 325°F (160°C).

Spray a foil-lined baking sheet with cooking spray. Arrange pork on prepared baking sheet and bake in preheated oven for 20 minutes.

⁂ "Hotty" Lamb Chops

1 lb	lean lamb chops	450 g
2 tbsp	water	30 mL
1 tbsp	ground cinnamon	15 mL
1 tbsp	dry mustard	15 mL
	Salt and freshly ground black pepper	

Preheat oven to 350°F (180°C).

Line a baking sheet with foil and spray with cooking spray.

Brush lamb with water and rub with cinnamon, mustard, salt, and pepper.

Place lamb chops on prepared baking sheet and cook in preheated oven for approximately 20–30 minutes.

&. Moroccan Lamb

Makes 4–6 servings.

1	leg of lamb (4–5 lbs/1.8–2.3 kg)	1
½	bunch fresh parsley	½
½	bunch fresh coriander	½
10	cloves garlic	10
½ cup	olive oil	125 mL
2 tbsp	Dijon mustard	30 mL
2 tbsp	ground cumin	30 mL
	Salt and freshly ground black pepper	

Trim any fat from the lamb and put the lamb in an ovenproof dish.

Cut slits throughout the lamb ½ inch (1 cm) deep and let it sit while you are preparing the other ingredients.

In the meantime, grind the parsley, coriander, and garlic in a food processor or blender. Combine with the oil, mustard, cumin, salt, and pepper to make a paste.

Preheat oven to 350°F (180°C).

Fill the slits in the lamb with the paste and rub the rest over the lamb. Cover with aluminum foil and cook in the preheated oven for 45 minutes. Remove the foil and roast for another 15 minutes to allow the lamb to get crisp.

SIDE DISHES

✒ Mashed Cauli (You won't believe it's not mashed potatoes)

1	medium head cauliflower	1
1 tbsp	fat-free sour cream	15 mL
½ tsp	minced garlic	2 mL
⅛ tsp	chicken soup base or bouillon powder (or ½ tsp/2 mL salt)	0.5 mL
⅛ tsp	freshly ground black pepper Non-hydrogenated light margarine or butter-flavored cooking spray	0.5 mL

Break cauliflower into small pieces. Cook in boiling water for about 6 minutes, or until soft. Drain well and quickly pat cauliflower dry between several layers of paper towels.

In a blender or food processor, purée the hot cauliflower with the sour cream, garlic, chicken soup base, and pepper until almost smooth. Serve hot with salt, pepper, and light margarine to taste.

⊷ Basic Spaghetti Squash

1   spaghetti squash, halved lengthwise and seeded   1

Preheat oven to 375°F (190°C).

Line a baking sheet with foil and spray with cooking spray. Place squash cut side down on prepared baking sheet and bake for 30 minutes in preheated oven.

Remove from oven and let cool until manageable. Take a fork and scrape out pulp, making spaghetti-like strands.

OPTIONS
Below are some great ways to dress your spaghetti squash; I'll give you more options in Phase Two.

⊷ Simple Squash

Add salt, pepper, and non-hydrogenated light margarine (or butter-flavored cooking spray).

⊷ Faux Tomato Pasta Primavera

Add tomato sauce and veggies for a faux tomato pasta primavera.

⊷ Cinnamon Squash

Add garlic, cinnamon, Splenda, and olive oil for a deliciously sweet treat.

❧ Skinny Jicama

2 tsp	canola oil	10 mL
12 oz	jicama, peeled and julienned	340 g
1	clove garlic, minced	1
1	red bell pepper, cut into thin strips	1
⅛ tsp	sweet ot hot paprika	0.5 mL
⅛ tsp	salt	0.5 mL
⅛ tsp	freshly ground black pepper	0.5 mL
⅛ tsp	fresh or dried basil	0.5 mL

Heat oil in medium frying pan over medium heat. Add jicama, garlic, and red pepper. Add seasonings and sauté for about 5 minutes.

❧ Steamed Veggies

I find that the easiest way to steam veggies is in the microwave. Use a microwave-safe casserole dish (get a few different sizes, as they come in so handy). Place veggies (asparagus, green beans, broccoli, and cauliflower work well) in dish with a little water, salt, and pepper. Cover and microwave on high for about 3–5 minutes. Drain water and add spices, freshly squeezed lemon juice, olive oil, or non-hydrogenated light margarine to taste.

Try adding garlic and a little non-hydrogenated light margarine or olive oil to the water before microwaving to infuse the veggies with flavor.

❧ Roasted Veggies

Preheat oven to 450°F (230°C).

Line a baking sheet with foil and spray with cooking spray.

Toss veggies (onions, portobellos, asparagus, broccoli, cauliflower, etc.) in a marinade of your choice. I like to use low-fat Italian dressing with a little salt, pepper, and basil because it's so easy. You can also use balsamic vinegar with a touch of olive oil, salt, pepper, basil, and garlic, or soy sauce, rice wine vinegar, and sesame oil for an Asian twist.

Scatter veggies on baking sheet and bake in preheated oven for approximately 30 minutes.

DESERTS

❧ Fruit Sorbet

Makes 1 serving.

1 cup	frozen berries, partially thawed	250 mL
1 tbsp	lemon juice	15 mL
	Sugar substitute (Splenda or stevia) to taste	

Mix all ingredients in blender or food processor and enjoy immediately. You can also add fat-free, artificially sweetened yogurt for more creaminess. Or try adding a little sparkling water to the blender for a really cool and delicious treat.

SAMPLE 14-DAY MENU PLAN

- This is a sample plan. Follow it if you like, or simply use it as a guide.
- Drink water with meals as often as possible.
- Items in italics indicate that a recipe is provided in the preceding section.
- Remember all foods are Phase One–appropriate, so "yogurt," for instance, means fat-free and artificially sweetened.
- Never eat salad before a meal; always eat it with the main dish. It takes up room on the plate and prevents you from overeating higher-calorie side dishes.

Day 1

BREAKFAST
Coffee with skim milk
Basic Egg White Omelette with asparagus and mushrooms

SNACK
Green tea
Nectarine

LUNCH
Fat-free sliced deli turkey (about 3 oz/90 g) atop mixed salad greens with veggies of your choice, dressed with low-fat Italian dressing

SNACK
Carrot and celery sticks with low-fat ranch dip

DINNER
Small green salad, dressed with low-fat dressing of your choice
Tilapia Pockets
Green tea

SNACK
Yogurt

Day 2

BREAKFAST
Coffee with skim milk
Basic Smoothie

SNACK
Hard-cooked egg whites and tomatoes

LUNCH
Basic Tuna Salad, on its own or atop a mixed green salad with fat-free Italian dressing
Apple
Green tea

SNACK
Breakthrough Mushroom Soup

DINNER
Asian-Style Cucumber
"Hotty" Lamb Chops
Steamed Veggies

SNACK
Diet gelatin (e.g. diet Jell-O)

Day 3

BREAKFAST
Coffee with skim milk
Fat-free cottage cheese, mixed
with berries and sweetened
with Splenda

SNACK
2 tangerines

LUNCH
Cobb Salad
Green tea

SNACK
Basic Smoothie

DINNER
Cherry tomatoes with chopped
green bell pepper and cucum-
ber, dressed with *Basic Balsamic
Dressing*
Basic Fish with grilled veggies

SNACK
Grapefruit, sweetened with
Splenda mixed with cinnamon

Day 4

BREAKFAST
Coffee with skim milk
Basic Protein Shake

SNACK
Plum
Green tea

LUNCH
Fat-free deli meat (about
3 oz/90 g) dipped in hot
mustard
Carrots and celery sticks
Yogurt

SNACK
Breakthrough Mushroom Soup

DINNER
Warm Asian Chicken Salad
Diet Fudgsicle™

SNACK
Frozen grapes

Day 5

BREAKFAST
Coffee with skim milk
Basic Egg White Omelette with
Asparagus, Feta, and Olives

SNACK
Yogurt
Green tea

LUNCH
The Best Homemade Chicken
Soup
Apple

SNACK
Sugar snap peas and carrots

DINNER
Ginger Salmon
Skinny Jicama
Steamed asparagus

SNACK
Fruit Sorbet

Day 6

BREAKFAST
Coffee with skim milk
Low-fat chicken, turkey, or ham
bacon—3 slices
Basic Egg White Omelette
Honeydew and cantaloupe
slices

SNACK
Green tea

LUNCH
Greek Salad

SNACK
Yogurt

DINNER
Lean cut of steak, grilled or
barbecued
Mashed Cauli
Steamed Veggies

SNACK
Grapefruit, with Splenda mixed
with cinnamon

Day 7

BREAKFAST
Skim milk latte
Smoked salmon with sliced
onion, tomatoes, and cucumber

SNACK
Fresh fruit salad

LUNCH
Cobb Salad

SNACK
Yogurt

DINNER
Mixed green salad with light
dressing
Faux Tomato Pasta Primavera
with chicken (sauté chicken
with the tomato sauce and
veggies) (125 mL) Because
spaghetti squash is one of the
more caloric Phase One foods, I
recommend limiting yourself to
about ½ cup (125 mL) per
serving.

SNACK
Pear

Day 8

BREAKFAST
Coffee with skim milk
Basic Protein Shake

SNACK
Fat-free cottage cheese and
berries, sweetened with Splenda

LUNCH
Greek Salad with grilled chicken

SNACK
Apple
Green tea

DINNER
Poached Salmon
Roasted Veggies
Asian-Style Cucumber

SNACK
Diet Fudgsicle™

Day 9

BREAKFAST
Coffee with skim milk
Basic Egg White Omelette with herbs

SNACK
Pear
Green Tea

LUNCH
Basic Tuna Salad in *Iceberg Lettuce Wrap*
Tangerine

SNACK
Veggies with low-fat ranch dip

DINNER
Boneless, skinless chicken breast, sautéed or baked, spiced as you please
Cinnamon Squash (125 mL)
Because spaghetti squash is one of the more caloric Phase One foods, I recommend limiting yourself to about ½ cup (125 mL) per serving.
Steamed Asparagus

SNACK
Diet gelatin

Day 10

BREAKFAST
Coffee with skim milk
Basic Smoothie

SNACK
Green tea
Fresh fruit salad

LUNCH
Deli turkey, chicken, or ham atop mixed green salad with veggies and light dressing of your choice
Light hot chocolate

SNACK
Tofu Delight

DINNER
Breakthrough Mushroom Soup
Basic Fish
Steamed green beans

SNACK
Grapefruit, topped with Splenda mixed with cinnamon

Day 11

BREAKFAST
Coffee with skim milk
Basic Egg White Omelette with Asparagus, Feta, and Olives

SNACK
Apple
Green tea

LUNCH
Faux Tomato Pasta Primavera (125 mL) Because spaghetti squash is one of the more caloric Phase One foods, I recommend limiting yourself to about ½ cup (125 mL) per serving.

SNACK
3 hard-cooked egg whites, with sliced tomatoes, salt, and pepper

DINNER
Tuna Steaks
Coleslaw
Grilled Portobello Mushrooms

SNACK
Frozen grapes
Diet Fudgsicle™

Day 12

BREAKFAST
Coffee with skim milk
Basic Protein Shake

SNACK
Apple
Green tea

LUNCH
Poached Salmon
Mixed green salad

SNACK
Fat-free cottage cheese and berries, sweetened with Splenda

DINNER
"Hotty" Pork Tenderloin
Mashed Cauli
Green salad

SNACK
Yogurt

Day 13

BREAKFAST
Coffee with skim milk
Basic Egg White Omelette with Bacon and Green Onion

SNACK
Nectarine
Green tea

LUNCH
Cobb Salad

SNACK
Yogurt

DINNER
Tangy Tilapia
Mixed green salad

SNACK
Fruit Sorbet

Day 14

BREAKFAST
Coffee with skim milk
2 chicken sausages, baked in oven
Basic Egg White Omelette
Watermelon

SNACK
Green tea

LUNCH
Breakthrough Mushroom Soup
Fruit salad with cottage cheese

SNACK
Celery and carrot sticks

DINNER
Basic Fish
Cinnamon Squash (125 mL)
Because spaghetti squash is one of the more caloric Phase One foods, I recommend limiting yourself to about ½ cup (125 mL) per serving.
Spinach sautéed in olive oil with garlic, salt, pepper, and onions

SNACK
Frozen grapes
Diet Fudgsicle™

A WIDER SELECTION

After two weeks in Phase One, switch to this phase of the diet. Like Phase One, this phase will last two weeks. In this phase, more carbohydrates, such as whole-grain breads, cereals, beans, and legumes, are introduced. Also, you can now choose from a wider selection of cheeses, meats, and sauces. While the foods introduced in this phase are lower in the "fourth macronutrient," they still possess the proper "hotty" and hormonal effects. This means that, despite the lower water content, weight loss will continue, as metabolism and fat-loss hormones remain elevated. While you should still use Phase One foods to form the basis of your diet, you can now add up to three portions of Phase Two foods per day. No more than three portions per day though! Remember, these foods are lower in water, so the calories can quickly add up if you overdo it.

Starting on page 133 you will find a list of foods for you to enjoy now that you are in Phase Two. I have provided information on serving sizes so that you know what constitutes a single portion. As in Phase One, I then discuss each of the categories of foods individually, highlighting their various health benefits. I also offer tips on how to best use and buy these foods as well as on how to estimate portion sizes without having to rely on weights and measures (I mean, get serious!).

Following this information, you will find an extensive collection of Phase Two–appropriate recipes and a 14-day sample menu plan. Once again, you can either follow the plan exactly or simply refer to it for meal ideas.

Foods to Enjoy in Phase Two

While I don't want you weighing and measuring your foods for life, it is important to get a mental picture of what a single portion size looks like. So go get a measuring cup, bowl, tablespoon, and plate out of your cupboard. If you have a deck of cards and some dice handy, grab those as well. As you read which foods are appropriate for Phase Two and what constitutes a single portion of that food, measure that food item. Look carefully at how much a single portion size actually amounts to on your plate or in your bowl. *It is absolutely crucial that you do this experiment.* When I first learned this information, I actually used a measuring cup to serve the portion onto my plate or into my bowl. Please trust me—this small effort will benefit your waistline and health for life!

Food	A Portion Is
Bread—must have 100 per-cent stone-ground whole wheat, bran, oat hull fiber, oat bran, corn bran, or rye as ingredients. **Those with the terms "enriched white flour," "honey," or "molasses" on the ingredient list cannot be consumed. (see p. 136)**	Bread—1 slice Pita—½ pita Tortilla—1 small, ½ large Crackers—4
Cereal—100 percent bran, All-Bran, Bran Buds, Fibre 1, Fibre First, Multi-Bran and oatmeal (large-flake, slow-cooking oats, as opposed to the instant variety)	¾ cup (175 mL) dry
Starch—barley; whole wheat pasta; long-grain basmati or wild rice	½ cup (125 mL) cooked
Starchy veggies—Corn; sweet potato and yam; turnip; parsnip; low-fat/fat-free microwavable or air-popped popcorn	Corn—½ cup (125 mL) canned or 1 cob Sweet potato or yam—½ medium to large Turnip—1 Parsnip—1 medium Popcorn—3 cups (750 mL) popped

Food	A Portion Is
Dried beans and lentils—soybeans, chickpeas, lentils, lima beans, fava beans, black beans, navy beans, pinto beans; hummus	½ cup (125 mL) canned or cooked 2 tablespoons (30 mL) hummus
Nuts and seeds	Nuts—1 small handful, or about 8 nuts Seeds—1 tablespoon (15 mL)
Animal-source protein—This category includes all meat and egg products that didn't qualify as appropriate for Phase One. These protein sources are higher in fat, which means that they are usually lower in water.	Red meats not listed in Phase One—3 oz/85 g Hamburger patty—3 oz/85 g This is roughly the size of 2 McDonald's regular hamburger patties or ½ a typical restaurant's patty. Meatballs—3 oz (85 g); 2 large or 4 small Dark meat of chicken or turkey—3 oz (85 g) Duck—3 oz (85 g) Fatty deli meats—3 oz (85 g) (those not listed in Phase One) Bacon—2 strips Sausage—2 small or 1 large Weiner—1 Egg with yolk—2

Food	A Portion Is
Dairy–goat cheese and cream cheese; any hard cheeses; chocolate milk (continue to choose reduced-fat varieties of all dairy products to maximize weight loss)	Goat cheese and cream cheese—2 tablespoons (30 mL) Solid cheese—1 oz (30 g) Skim or partly-skimmed chocolate milk—1 cup (250 mL)
Fats—All oils that didn't qualify as appropriate for Phase One, (including full-fat salad dressings, butter, margarine, mayonnaise)	1 tablespoon (15 mL)
Extra—any condiments or sauces that weren't listed in Phase One	See page 140

Carbohydrates

This category includes the breads, cereals, and starches listed in "Foods to Enjoy in Phase Two."

TIPS

⇨ To avoid unwanted added sugar, always buy oatmeal plain and flavor it yourself. I like to add cinnamon mixed with sugar substitute, berries (fresh or thawed), and some slivered almonds. Try it cold with some skim milk; it's a wonderful alternative to prepared cereals.

⇨ Always buy large-flake, slow-cooked oats and not the "instant" or "quick-cooking oats" variety. Instant varieties have been altered to make them less "hotty," so we burn fewer calories when we digest them.

⇨ Oatmeal and barley are extremely high in soluble fiber and are therefore "hotty," helping stabilize blood sugar and insulin levels. Diets high in soluble fiber help prevent diabetes and high cholesterol, two of the biggest risk factors for strokes and heart attack. Remember, a bowl of oatmeal or barley a day helps keep the cardiologist away!

⇨ Do not buy breads, pitas, cereals, and crackers that have the terms "sugar," "enriched white flour," "honey," or "molasses" in the ingredient lists. These are not "hotty." Most often, the shorter the list of ingredients, the better!

⇨ The coarser the bread or cracker, the more insoluble fiber it contains and the more our bodies have to work to break it down. In this way we can dispose of many calories unused. These items are "hotty" and lead to more stable insulin levels. If you are not used to eating foods high in insoluble fiber, start slowly with these foods to allow your gut time to adjust to the increased bulk.

⇨ Diets high in insoluble fiber help fight constipation, diverticulitis, and colon cancer. Remember to drink plenty of water with high-fiber foods to ensure regularity.

Starchy Vegetables

These veggies are higher in carbohydrate content and lower in water than those listed in Phase One. However, they are excellent sources of fiber and nutrients. I frequently choose from this category when selecting my Phase Two food choices for the day.

TIPS

⇨ Eat the skin with your sweet potato and yams. The skin has loads of fiber that will slow the digestion and absorption of the sugar contained within the potato.

⇨ Top sweet potatoes with some cinnamon mixed with Splenda or stevia for a deliciously sweet and healthy treat.

⇨ Corn is wonderful eaten alone or sprinkled into salads. Do not buy creamed varieties or those with added sugar.

⇨ Popcorn is an excellent snack as it is high in water-loving fiber. In the mood for a sweet snack? Pop some popcorn and then lightly drizzle it with liquid honey, just enough to get it a little sticky. Then sprinkle it with cinnamon, Splenda, some almonds or pecan halves, and bake it in the oven for a few minutes. Voila, candy corn that is "hotty" and won't spike insulin levels!

Plant-Source Protein

This category includes dried beans and lentils as well as nuts and seeds.

TIPS

⇨ Dried beans and lentils are exceptionally good sources of soluble fiber. These foods are very filling as they attract water in our stomachs and form gels. Therefore, a ½-cup (125 mL) serving is very filling. The soluble fiber contained within dried beans and lentils has been shown to help lower cholesterol. Sprinkle them into pasta sauces and salads or use them to make deliciously filling and healthy soups! Always rinse canned varieties with cold water to remove excess salt.

⇨ Nuts and seeds are excellent sources of protein and fiber. However, they are high in "water-hating" fat and low in water, so they can be high in calories. If you stick to the recommended portions, you can reap the tasty benefits without packing on pounds.

⇨ I give nuts and seeds a guest appearance rather than a starring role in my meals. For instance, I add a small handful of toasted pine nuts to salads, a small handful of slivered almonds to green beans, 1 tablespoon (30 mL) of poppy seeds to fish, etc.

⇨ Nut-based spreads such as peanut butter and Nutella are high in sugar, low in water, high in fat, and less "hotty" than the actual nuts themselves. These items are not appropriate for Phase Two and best avoided when trying to lose weight.

⇨ Men, eat your pumpkin seeds! An association has been found between pumpkin seeds and protection against prostate cancer.

⇨ Go nuts for almonds. They are an excellent source of disease-fighting fiber and minerals. I buy slivered almonds and toast them in the oven (400°F for 3–5 minutes) on a baking sheet. I love to sprinkle them on salads, veggies, oatmeal, and fruit.

Animal-Source Protein

Recall that one portion of most meats is 3 ounces (85 g). To help visualize this amount, use the following "card trick." A 3-ounce portion of meat is roughly the size and thickness of a deck of playing cards. Put a deck of cards on your plate. Is this your typical serving size? Probably not! If you have a cut of meat that's twice that thickness, two decks of cards stacked, as I often do, just count it as two portions. If it's twice the thickness and takes up a little more room, count it as three portions. If you order a 9-ounce (255 g) steak at a restaurant, and eat it all, you've just eaten three portions. Keep a deck of cards on your kitchen table for the first few weeks that you're on the Hershberg Diet. Each time you eat a higher-fat cut of meat, use it to help estimate your portion size.

This card trick works for almost all kinds of meat. Each time you eat dark meat from a chicken or turkey (remember, the white meat is low in fat, so it qualifies for Phase One), consider how many slices you could fit in the deck of cards. Having a hamburger patty or meatballs? Think about the size of a deck of cards and judge your portion size based on it. Eventually, you'll inherently know the correct portion sizes. For deli meats, 3 ounces is roughly equivalent to 85 grams. I often ask the deli server to individually wrap 3-ounce portions, which makes estimates unnecessary.

All animal-source proteins (meats and whole eggs) are considered appropriate for Phase Two because proteins are "hotty" (remember, protein requires a lot of work to break down) and do not cause our blood sugar and insulin levels to spike. However, I suggest that you stick to the lower-fat meats introduced in Phase One as often as possible, saving your three portions of Phase Two foods for the other healthier choices listed above, such as nuts, seeds, dried beans, and high-fiber carbohydrates. I tend to eat the Phase Two fatty meats only when I am out at a restaurant. I find that the lower-fat Phase One varieties taste just as good and I know that they are certainly better for my health. However, so long as you stick to the rules, you can choose however you like and still lose weight!

There is one last category that I must mention: extras.

Extras

Extras are any condiments or sauces that weren't listed in Phase One, e.g., honey, teriyaki, cranberry sauce, ketchup, relish, BBQ sauce, etc.

I didn't include extras in the list of Phase Two–appropriate foods because it is far too tedious to measure out portions of condiments and sauces. However, you can include any sauce or condiment that you like in Phase Two and you needn't worry about counting them into your three portions of Phase Two foods per day. Remember that most condiments and sauces are high in either sugar and/or fat, but they do add zip to healthy Phase One and Phase Two foods. So simply be mindful of the types and quantity that you are using, and try to use Phase One spices, sauces, condiments, and low-fat dressings in their place as often as possible. A good rule of thumb is to not use more than 2 tablespoons (30 mL) of sauces or condiments per meal and to avoid any sauce that looks creamy or, even worse, has the word "sweet," "rich," or "cream" as a part of its name. These sauces can derail even the most committed dieter's efforts.

PHASE TWO

APPROPRIATE RECIPES

Now that you are familiar with the various Phase Two–appropriate foods and their respective portion sizes, let's review some delicious and easy-to-make recipes that incorporate these items. Again, a 14-day sample menu plan will follow.

Now that you are in Phase Two, you have a lot more foods to choose from. You can now jazz up some of the recipe ideas introduced in Phase One. For instance, you can add any type of cheese to omelettes (we were limited to feta in Phase One) and nuts and seeds to veggies and fish, plus you now have many more sauces to choose from. Just remember to have no more than three portions per day of foods introduced in Phase Two.

BREAKFAST

ᕽ Mexican Omelette
Makes 1 serving.

Prepare *Basic Egg White Omelette* as in Phase One. When cooked, remove lid and add up to ½ cup (125 mL) black beans and up to ¼ cup (60 mL) grated light cheddar cheese. Cover for about 1 minute so the steam will warm the dish up and melt the cheese. Remove lid and top with salsa. Delicious!

ᕽ The Very Best Cereal
Makes 1 serving.

½ cup (125 mL) oats + ¼ cup (60 mL) Bran Buds or Fibre 1
    (total = ¾ cup/175 mL = 1 Phase Two portion)

1   small handful (about 1 oz/30 g, or 8 whole nuts)   1
      slivered almonds (1 Phase Two portion)
      Fresh berries
      Skim milk
      Splenda, mixed with cinnamon

Add the oats, fiber cereal, almonds and berries to skim milk. Sweeten with Splenda mixed with cinnamon to taste. Eat cold. This counts as two of your servings of Phase Two foods per day, but it's worth it. It's delicious and excellent for your health.

LUNCH AND DINNER

SALADS

❧ Jicama, Orange, and Almond Salad

Makes 4 servings.

1	jicama (1½ pound/680 g)	1
2–3 cups	fresh orange sections	500–750 mL
¼ tsp	salt	1 mL
1	dash chili powder	
4 oz	slivered almonds (about 4 small handfuls)	115 g
3 tbsp	chopped fresh cilantro	45 mL

Peel and slice jicama; slice into 2-inch (5 cm) strips. Toss with the orange sections, salt, and chili powder. Refrigerate.

Preheat oven to 400°F (200°C).

Five minutes before serving, bake slivered almonds on a baking sheet in preheated oven for about 3–5 minutes, being careful that they don't burn (1 oz. of slivered almonds equals approximately one Phase Two portion). Scatter almonds over salad and garnish with cilantro.

❧ Caesar Salad

Use portions of the following ingredients to taste, but remember that 1 oz (30 g) of cheese equals one Phase Two portion.

SALAD

> Romaine lettuce, chopped
> Cherry tomatoes
> Bacon bits (it is best to use chopped low-fat chicken or turkey bacon)
> Freshly grated Parmesan cheese

Toss desired amounts of lettuce, tomatoes, bacon bits, and cheese in a large bowl.

DRESSING

¼ cup	fat-free mayonnaise	60 mL
¼ cup	fat-free plain yogurt (or use ½ cup of either mayo or yogurt)	60 mL
2 tbsp	freshly squeezed lemon juice	30 mL
1 tsp	olive oil	5 mL
1 tsp	white wine vinegar	5 mL
1 tsp	Dijon mustard	5 mL
1 tsp	Worcestershire sauce	5 mL
2	garlic cloves, minced	2
¼ cup	freshly grated Parmesan (equivalent to 2 oz/60 g) (optional)	60 mL

Mix mayonnaise, yogurt, lemon juice, oil, vinegar, Worcestershire sauce, garlic, and cheese.

Pour over salad, toss, and enjoy! This is great topped with grilled chicken breast.

(If you don't want to make your own dressing, buy a low-fat Caesar dressing and dilute with white wine vinegar and lemon juice.)

∾ Apple and Walnut Salad

Makes 4 servings.

SALAD

¼ cup	apple cider vinegar	60 mL
¼ cup	Splenda mixed with cinnamon	60 mL
1–2	green apples, cored and sliced	1–2
1 cup	walnut halves or pecan halves (approx. ¼ cup/ 60 mL, or one small handful, per plate, which is one Phase Two portion)	250 mL
4 cups	mixed greens	1L
1	cucumber, sliced	1
1	red bell pepper, sliced	1
	Cooking spray	
2 tbsp	Liquid honey	30 mL

DRESSING

3 tbsp	canola oil	45 mL
2 tbsp	fat-free plain yogurt	30 mL
½ cup	freshly grated Parmesan cheese (2 tbsp/30 mL = 1 oz/30 g per person, which is one Phase Two portion)	125 mL

In a small bowl, combine vinegar and Splenda mixed with cinnamon. Pour over apples and let soak.

Combine mixed greens, cucumber, and red pepper and set aside.

Microwave liquid honey for about 30 seconds. Reserving liquid, drain apples and place on a large plate with the walnuts. Drizzle both with the honey—just to make them sticky—and toss with Splenda mixed with cinnamon.

Preheat oven to 400°F (200°C). Line a cookie sheet with aluminum foil. Spray with cooking spray and scatter walnuts and apples on top. Bake in preheated oven for about 3–5 minutes, watching carefully so they don't burn. Remove from oven and let cool.

Meanwhile, add canola oil and yogurt to reserved soaking liquid. Whisk, adding honey to sweeten to taste.

Toss dressing with salad and scatter apples, walnuts, and Parmesan over.

✑ Better Than Eggplant Parmesan

Makes 8 servings.

2 tbsp	olive oil	30 mL
1	medium eggplant	1
1 cup	chopped green bell pepper	250 mL
1	can (8 oz/228 mL) tomato sauce	1
¼ tsp	dried oregano, crumbled	1 mL
3–4	fresh basil leaves (or 1 tsp/5 mL dry basil)	3–4
3–4	cloves garlic, minced	3–4
½ tsp	fine sea salt	2 mL
¼ tsp	freshly ground black pepper	1 mL
1 cup	sliced green onions (include green tops)	250 mL
½ cup	sliced olives (canned or fresh), divided	125 mL
2 cups	shredded low-fat mozzarella cheese, divided	500 mL

Cut unpeeled eggplant into ½-inch (1 cm) cubes; set aside. Coat a large microwave-safe dish with olive oil. Microwave, uncovered, on high for 30 seconds to heat oil. Add eggplant and green pepper; mix to coat with the oil. Cover loosely with waxed paper. Microwave on high for 4 minutes.

Combine tomato sauce with oregano, basil, garlic, salt, pepper, green onions, and ⅓ cup (75 mL) of the olives. Stir into eggplant mixture. Mix in 1½ cups (375 mL) of the cheese. Microwave, uncovered, on high for 8–10 minutes. Sprinkle with remaining olives and ½ cup (125 mL) cheese.

Let stand for 3 to 4 minutes before serving.

Each serving contains one Phase Two portion.

⮿ Salmon Patties

Makes 2 servings.

1	can (14.75 oz/418 g) salmon	1
2	egg whites	2
1 tsp	freshly squeezed lemon juice	5 mL
½	medium onion, chopped	½
1 tsp	freshly ground black pepper	5 mL
¾ cup	oats (1 Phase Two serving)	175 mL
2 tbsp	canola or vegetable oil	30 mL

Empty the can of salmon with juice into a large mixing bowl and remove bones. Add egg whites and lemon juice. Stir well and add onion, pepper, and oats. (The oats should absorb the moisture, and you may need less than ¾ cup.) Form into 6 patties and set aside.

Heat oil in a nonstick frying pan and cook patties for approximately 4 minutes per side, until outside is browned and center is no longer cool.

Alternatively, you can bake the patties in the oven to eliminate the need for oil. Preheat oven to 400°F (200°C). Line a cookie sheet with foil and spray well with cooking spray. Place patties on foil and bake in preheated oven for 10 minutes, flip, and cook for another 10 minutes. They will be brown and warm inside when done.

Six patties equals one Phase Two portion (for the ¾ cup oats). I find that 3 patties is a good portion size, so you only have to count this as half of a Phase Two portion.

OPTIONS

✍ Tuna Patties

Substitute tuna for salmon, using the same recipe and procedure as for *Salmon Patties*.

✍ Meatballs

Substitute lean ground chicken, turkey, or beef in *Salmon Patties*. Instead of forming into patties, form into meatballs. These taste great topped with a sweet tomato sauce. To make a healthy, sweet-tasting tomato sauce, heat a can of plain tomato sauce and add spices and Splenda to sweeten to taste.

❧ Baked Fish

Makes 4 servings.

4	4 oz fish fillets (tilapia, halibut, sole, or cod)	4
½ cup	fresh mushrooms, sliced	125 mL
1	green bell pepper, seeded and cut into 1-inch (2.5 cm) pieces	1
1	cooking onion, sliced	1
2 tbsp	chicken broth or water	30 mL
1 cup	salsa	250 mL
½ cup	freshly grated Parmesan (4 oz/125 g)	125 mL

Spray a large microwave-safe dish with cooking spray. Layer fish along bottom and add mushrooms, pepper, onion, and broth.

Microwave, covered, with a slight opening for steam to vent on high for 5 minutes. Drain juices. Spoon salsa over the vegetables and cook for another minute or so, until salsa is heated. Top with Parmesan.

Count 1 serving (1 piece of fish) as one Phase Two portion (2 tbsp/ 30 mL parmesan = 1 oz).

⨍ Squash Lasagna

Makes approximately 8 servings.

1	large spaghetti squash	1
	Store-bought tomato sauce of your choice	
1 cup	shredded partly-skimmed mozzarella cheese (8oz/250 g), divided	250 mL
½ cup	Freshly grated Parmesan (4 oz/125 g)	125 mL
½ cup	sliced black olives	125 mL
1 lb	sliced mushrooms	500 g
1	eggplant, sliced thinly	1

Make *Basic Spaghetti Squash* (see recipes, page 120) or pierce a few holes in the squash and microwave on high for approximately 15 minutes. Let it cool and then cut lengthwise, removing seeds. Scrape spaghetti squash with fork to form strands like spaghetti.

Preheat oven to 350°F (180°C). Spray a 9- × 13-inch (3L) ovenproof dish with cooking spray. Spoon in tomato sauce to lightly cover the bottom of the dish. Layer spaghetti squash over and pat down. Pour in another layer of tomato sauce. Next place a layer of eggplant, then a layer of shredded mozzarella cheese (½ cup/125 mL). Place another layer of squash on top, and cover with tomato sauce. On top place a layer of mushrooms and a layer of mozzarella cheese (½ cup). Sprinkle Parmesan on top. Bake in preheated oven for 30 minutes.

Count 1 serving of lasagna as 1½ Phase Two portions.

Note: You can substitute sautéed extra-lean ground beef for the veggies (mushrooms, eggplant, and olives) if you want to create a meat lasagna.

✍ Barley with Mushrooms

So good for a cold winter day!
Makes 4 servings.

2 tbsp	oil (vegetable, canola or olive)	30 mL
1	medium onion, chopped	1
½ lb	mushrooms, sliced	225 g
1 cup	barley	250 mL
	Salt and freshly ground black pepper to taste	
2½ cups	vegetable broth, boiling	625 mL

Preheat oven to 350°F (180°C).

Heat oil in a large frying pan. Sauté onion, mushrooms, barley, salt, and pepper. Stir frequently until barley is lightly browned. Place in a large casserole dish (about 8 cups/2 L) and stir in broth.

Cover and bake in preheated oven for approximately 1 hour. (If barley is too firm when all liquid is absorbed add additional ½ cup (125 mL) boiling water and bake another 15 minutes.)

Count ½ cup (125 mL) as 1 serving, which should be counted as one Phase Two portion.

14-DAY SAMPLE MENU PLAN

- This is a sample plan. Follow it if you like, or simply use it as a guide.
- Drink water with meals as often as possible.
- Items in italics indicate that a recipe was listed in Phase One or Two.
- Notice that there are no more than three servings of Phase Two–appropriate foods per day
- Never eat salad before a meal; always eat it with the main dish.

Day 1

BREAKFAST
Coffee with skim milk
Mexican Omelette

SNACK
Pear
Green tea

LUNCH
Half a whole wheat pita, filled
with fat-free deli turkey, alfalfa
sprouts, sliced cucumbers, and
mustard
Yogurt

SNACK
Veggies with fat-free ranch dip

DINNER
Mixed green salad with low-fat
dressing of your choice
Baked Fish

SNACK
Frozen grapes, 1–2 handfuls

Day 2

BREAKFAST
Coffee with skim milk
The Very Best Cereal

SNACK
Yogurt

LUNCH
Greek Salad with chicken

SNACK
Apple

DINNER
Skinless, boneless breast of
chicken, baked or sautéed
Steamed asparagus
Apple and Walnut Salad

SNACK
Diet gelatin

Day 3

BREAKFAST

Coffee with skim milk

Hot oatmeal (Mix ¾ cup old-fashioned oats with 1½ cups (375 mL) water; heat in microwave according to package directions. Sweeten with Splenda mixed with cinnamon.)

SNACK

Fat-free cottage cheese, mixed with fruit and sweetened with Splenda

LUNCH

Mixed green salad with ½ cup (125 mL) chickpeas and assorted veggies of your choice. Dress with low-fat dressing.

Apple

SNACK

Breakthrough Mushroom Soup

DINNER

Ginger Salmon

Steamed green beans (I like to bake slivered almonds in the oven for about 3 minutes and add them to the beans. Remember, for each handful of nuts, count one Phase Two portion. Top with salt, pepper, and either olive oil, non-hydrogenated light margarine, or butter spray.)

SNACK

Cherries (about 10)

Diet Fudgsicle™

Day 4

BREAKFAST
Coffee with skim milk
Basic Smoothie

SNACK
3 hard-cooked egg whites

LUNCH
Basic Tuna Salad, mixed with tomatoes, cucumbers, and salad greens
Fresh fruit salad

SNACK
Carrot and celery sticks

DINNER
Caesar Salad
Squash Lasagna

SNACK
Diet hot chocolate

Day 5

BREAKFAST
Coffee and skim milk
Basic Egg White Omelette with Asparagus, Feta, and Olives

SNACK
Banana

LUNCH
Turkey sandwich (use fat-free deli turkey and place between two pieces of Phase Two—appropriate bread. I like to add sliced cucumbers, tomatoes and hot mustard to mine.)
Orange

SNACK
3 cups light popcorn, with butter-flavored spray and sprinkled with Splenda mixed with cinnamon

DINNER
Mixed green salad
Tilapia Pockets

SNACK
Diet Fudgsicle™

Day 6

BREAKFAST
Coffee with skim milk
Basic Protein Shake

SNACK
Green tea

LUNCH
Warm Asian Chicken Salad

SNACK
Slices of fresh fruit

DINNER
Basic Fish
Barley with Mushrooms
(½ cup/125 mL)
Steamed asparagus

SNACK
Fruit sorbet

Day 7

BREAKFAST
Coffee with skim milk
The Very Best Cereal

SNACK
Tangerine

LUNCH
Poached Salmon
Mixed green salad

SNACK
3 cups (750 mL) low-fat
popcorn

DINNER
Greek Salad
"Hotty" Lamb Chops
Portobello mushrooms, mari-
nated in low-fat Italian dressing,
balsamic vinegar, salt, pepper,
and basil and then sautéed

SNACK
Frozen grapes, 1–2 handfuls

Day 8

BREAKFAST
Coffee with skim milk
Basic Egg White Omelette
One piece toast, with fat-free
cream cheese

SNACK
Green tea
Yogurt

LUNCH
Mixed green salad with veggies,
grilled chicken, 1 tablespoon
(15 mL) sunflower seeds, and
light Italian dressing

SNACK
Apple

DINNER
Sliced turkey breast, ½ cup
(125 mL) wild rice, and steamed
broccoli

SNACK
Diet gelatin

Day 9

BREAKFAST
Coffee with skim milk
Two 6-oz (175 mL) fat-free,
artificially sweetened yogurts

SNACK
A small handful mixed nuts
Orange

LUNCH
*The Best Homemade Chicken
Soup*
Mixed green salad

SNACK
Partly-skimmed chocolate milk

DINNER
Lean steak
Green beans, with toasted
almonds
Coleslaw

SNACK
Frozen grapes, 1–2 handfuls

Day 10

BREAKFAST
Coffee with skim milk
The Very Best Cereal

SNACK
Green tea
Plum

LUNCH
Fat-free deli turkey meat,
dipped in hot mustard
Yogurt
Carrot and celery sticks

SNACK
Breakthrough Mushroom Soup

DINNER
Basic Fish
Moroccan Lamb
Cucumbers and tomatoes,
tossed in a light vinaigrette

SNACK
Nectarine

Day 11

BREAKFAST
Coffee with skim milk
Basic Egg White Omelette

SNACK
2 plums

LUNCH
Cobb Salad with chicken

SNACK
Veggies and fat-free ranch dip

DINNER
Caesar salad with grilled
chicken

SNACK
3 cups (750 mL) light popcorn

Day 12

BREAKFAST
Coffee with skim milk
Basic Protein Shake

SNACK
Green tea
Orange

LUNCH
Half a whole wheat pita, filled
with *Basic Tuna Salad*, sliced
cucumber, and alfalfa sprouts
Yogurt

SNACK
Grapefruit, topped with
Splenda mixed with cinnamon

DINNER
Apple and Walnut Salad
Lean steak
Steamed asparagus

SNACK
Diet gelatin

Day 13

BREAKFAST
Coffee with skim milk
Cottage cheese, mixed with
fruit

SNACK
Green tea

LUNCH
Mixed green salad
Salmon Patties

SNACK
Veggies and low-fat ranch dip

DINNER
Caesar salad
Sautéed chicken and veggies in
tomato sauce, served over ½ cup
(125 mL) whole wheat pasta

SNACK
Fruit sorbet

Day 14

BREAKFAST
Coffee with skim milk
2 slices low-fat turkey, chicken,
or ham bacon
Basic Egg White Omelette
Slices of fruit

SNACK
Green tea

LUNCH
Fat-free deli turkey atop a
mixed salad with light dressing

SNACK
3 cups (750 mL) light popcorn

DINNER
Lean grilled or broiled steak
Roasted Veggies
Mashed Cauli

SNACK
Diet hot chocolate

CONGRATULATIONS

You've made it to Phase Three—the final phase for weight loss! You will remain in this phase until you reach your goal weight. You should be looking and feeling great. You've probably lost a noticeable amount of weight as well as having improved your blood chemistry and overall health. You'll be delighted to know that in this phase you can eat any food you like. That's right! No food is off-limits.

Phase Three foods are traditionally thought of as bad for weight loss; they are low in water, burn few calories in their breakdown, and encourage a fat-storing hormonal effect. These foods consist mainly of "white foods," like white bread, potatoes, rice, pasta, fries, and bakery products; snack foods like chips, pretzels, cookies, and granola bars; and junk food like chocolate bars, candy, pop, ice cream, etc. The problem is that these are the foods we love! In this phase you will learn a strategy so that you can indulge in these delicious items without destroying your weight loss and health goals.

Phase Three Strategy

1. 1000 Calories a Week

Because Phase Three foods are costly to your diet, you must keep track of how much you eat of them. The easiest way to do this is with the help of the calorie information on nutrition labels.

To be able to eat Phase Three foods while still losing weight, you must restrict yourself to a limit of no more than 1000 calories per week of them. It's as simple as that. I suggest that you always round off to the nearest multiple of 100. For example, if the nutrition label on a chocolate bar says one bar equals 320 calories, and you eat the entire bar, that's fine; you must count 300 calories, so now you have 700 calories left for the week. *Remember, you can still eat as many Phase One foods as you like, plus your three portions of Phase Two foods per day.* If you look at the "7-Day sample Menu Plan" that starts on page 173, you'll see just how easy this is to do.

If you absolutely detest counting and can't keep track of the day of the week, don't worry. However, you must develop a system that limits the amount of Phase Three foods you consume. If you don't, you'll gain weight. Maybe you want to choose a "cheat" day to treat yourself. Maybe you should eat Phase Three foods only on special occasions. I find that for me the best system is that of 1000 calories a week, but it's up to you. If you find that weight loss slows in Phase Three or that you are being a little too liberal with these foods, just skip back to Phase One for a week or two until you're back on track.

2. Splurging Tips

These tips include strategies we can use to trick our bodies into thinking that we've consumed a healthier, higher-water food than we have. We are trying to improve the water ratio as well as the "hotty" and hormonal effect of Phase Three foods.

First, we must find a way to increase the water content and calorie-burning potential of the food. If we consume Phase Three foods with a full glass of cold water or green tea, we accomplish this goal quite easily. Recall that in addition to being obviously high in water, cold water and green tea are "hotty." When we drink them, our body is encouraged to burn calories.

Our second goal involves finding a way to improve the hormonal effect; we want to slow the absorption of sugar into our blood. Again, this is easily accomplished. We simply have to eat Phase Three foods with or immediately following a Phase One or Phase Two food, which will tend to have more protein, fiber, or fat. All three of these substances slow the rate at which we digest and absorb sugar, thus improving the net hormonal effect. Alternatively, you may choose to eat the Phase Three food along with a fish oil or flaxseed oil supplement (limit supplements to two per day). This will achieve the same effect.

Let's review the Phase Three strategy:
1. Any food that was not listed in Phase One or Phase Two is considered a Phase Three food. Most often, these are "white foods," snack foods, or junk foods.
2. You may eat up to 1000 calories per week of Phase Three foods. Note the calories per serving size that you are about to eat, round this number to the closest multiple of 100, and keep track of this amount. Most Phase Three foods are processed snack-type foods that come with nutrition labels, so this task is relatively easy to do. For further help, I have provided estimates of the calorie

counts associated with commonly consumed Phase Three foods in the chart that follows. Whenever the nutrition label is available, though, use it instead.

3. You cannot carry over leftover calories to subsequent weeks. If you do not eat your total allowed amount, you will lose weight a little more quickly!

4. Consume foods with a full glass of cold water or green tea. This increases the water content and makes the food more "hotty."

5. Consume foods along with or immediately following meals of Phase One or Phase Two foods. If you want to have the food on its own as a snack, simply take one fish oil or flaxseed oil supplement along with the food.

Examples of Foods to Enjoy in Phase Three

(**Note:** Whenever nutrition labels are available, use them instead.)

Food	Serving	Calorie Count
BREADS with ingredients such as enriched white flour, sugar, honey, molasses, or fine-ground, which don't qualify as appropriate for Phase Two		
Sliced bread	1 piece	100

Food	Serving	Calorie Count
Pita	1 medium	200
Tortilla wrap	1 large	200
Bagel	1 whole	300
Pancake	1 large or 2 small	200
Waffle	1 large or 3 small	300
Dinner roll	1	100
Muffin	1 large or 2 mini	400
Low-fat muffin	1 large	300
Croissant	1	300
Hamburger/hotdog bun	1	200
Cereals (other than those suitable for Phase Two)	1 cup	200
Crackers	4	100
SIDE DISHES		
Baked potato	1	200
Pasta	1 cup (250 mL), cooked	200
Rice	1 cup (250 mL), cooked	200
Sushi rice	6 maki rolls	100

Food	Serving	Calorie Count
Fried rice	1 cup (250 mL), cooked	300
Couscous	1 cup (250 mL), cooked	200
French fries	¼ plate portion, or about 20 fries	400
SNACKS AND DESSERTS		
Potato chips	1 snack size bag (2.6 oz/75 g)	400
Pretzels	1 snack size bag (2.0 oz/60 g)	200
Movie theater popcorn	1 small bag	600
Cookies	1 large or 2 small	100
Chocolate bar	1	300
Granola bar	1	200
Breakfast bar	1	200
Doughnut	1	300
Cake, iced	1 piece	400
Pie	1 piece	400
CANDY		
Licorice	2 pieces	100

Food	Serving	Calorie Count
Jelly beans, gummies, etc.	10 pieces	100
Hard candies	5 pieces	100
Dried fruit	1 handful	100
COLD DESSERTS		
Regular ice cream	½ cup (125 mL)	300
Low-fat or fat-free ice cream	½ cup (125 mL)	100
Sherbet, sorbet, or milk-free gelati	½ cup (125 mL)	100
Gelati containing milk	½ cup (125 mL)	200
Low-fat or fat-free frozen yogurt	½ cup (125 mL)	100
Milkshakes	1 (about 12 fluid oz/355 ml)	400
DRINKS		
Cola	1 can (12 oz/355 mL)	100
Juice	1 cup (250 mL)	100

On the following page, I have provided you with a 7-day sample menu plan to show you what a typical week could look like in Phase Three of the diet.

7-DAY SAMPLE MENU PLAN

- *Drink water with meals as often as possible, as we did in the other phases.*

Day 1

BREAKFAST
¾ cup (175 mL) plain, large-flake oatmeal, topped with Splenda mixed with cinnamon, and blueberries
Coffee with skim milk

SNACK
Apple

LUNCH
Turkey sandwich: low-fat (preferably low-sodium) deli turkey on two slices of 100 percent stone-ground whole wheat bread, with tomato, pickle, and mustard
Tangerine
Chocolate-coated granola bar (**200 calories**), consumed with a full 8-oz (250 mL) glass of ice water

SNACK
Carrot and celery sticks with fat-free ranch dip

DINNER
Seasoned boneless, skinless chicken breast
Grilled eggplant, peppers, and mushrooms, topped with olive oil and balsamic vinegar
Salad topped with olives, cucumbers, and tomatoes, sprinkled with feta cheese, with olive oil and balsamic vinegar dressing
Water

SNACK
Grapefruit, topped with Splenda mixed with cinnamon

Day 1 count of Phase Three foods = 200 calories

Day 2

BREAKFAST

Fat-free cottage cheese, topped with fruit

SNACK

Skim milk latte with cinnamon

LUNCH

Chicken breast, grilled
Salad of spinach, cucumber, tomatoes, 1 tablespoon (15 mL) sunflower seeds, and light Italian dressing
Water

SNACK

Apple

DINNER

½ cup (125 mL) whole wheat pasta, topped with vegetarian sauce made from mushrooms, onions, garlic, tomato sauce, ½ cup (125 mL) chickpeas, olive oil, and spices
Caesar Salad
Diet pop

SNACK

Fat-free, artificially sweetened yogurt

**Day 2 count of Phase Three foods = 0
Cumulative count of Phase Three foods = 200 calories**

Day 3

BREAKFAST
The Very Best Cereal
Coffee with skim milk

SNACK
Fat-free, artificially sweetened
yogurt

LUNCH
Tuna Salad in half a whole
wheat pita
Salad of lettuce, beets, cucumber, and tomato, topped with
low-fat Italian dressing

SNACK
Sugar snap peas and celery
sticks
Green tea

DINNER
Lean steak, with all visible fat
trimmed
Grilled portobello mushrooms,
brushed with olive oil and balsamic vinegar
Steamed green beans

SNACK
Frozen grapes, 1–2 handfuls

**Day 3 count of Phase Three
foods = 0**
**Cumulative count of Phase
Three foods = 200 calories**

Day 4

BREAKFAST
Apple
Coffee with skim milk

SNACK
Granola bar (**200 calories**)
Green tea and flaxseed oil
supplement

LUNCH
Half a whole wheat pita,
filled with 2 tbsp (30 mL)
hummus, alfalfa sprouts,
cucumber, turkey deli meat,
and a few sliced olives
3 mini chocolates (**100
calories**)

SNACK
Decaffeinated skim milk latte
Plum

DINNER
Ginger Salmon
Spinach salad with a small
handful of toasted pine nuts
and cherry tomatoes, with low-
fat strawberry dressing

SNACK
Fat-free, artificially sweetened
yogurt

**Day 4 count of Phase Three
foods = 300 calories
Cumulative count of Phase
Three foods = 500 calories**

Day 5

BREAKFAST
Fat-free cottage cheese with honeydew, cantaloupe, and a small handful of slivered almonds
Coffee with skim milk

SNACK
Banana
Green tea

LUNCH
Chicken deli meat atop large salad of mixed greens, cucumber, tomato, peppers, broccoli, and 1 tablespoon (15 mL) sunflower seeds, with light dressing
Diet iced tea

SNACK
Nectarine

DINNER
(This in an example of something that you could order at a restaurant.)
Salad with roasted red peppers, mushrooms, and about 2 tablespoons (30 mL) goat cheese (ask for dressing on side and use sparingly; I often ask for balsamic vinegar and use it instead of the oily dressing)
Baked trout in lemon-dill sauce
Asparagus
Steamed spinach instead of the rice that the trout was supposed to be served with (most restaurants will substitute veggies for other side dishes if you ask)
2 glasses of red wine
½ slice decadent chocolate cake
(400 ÷ 2 = 200 calories)

Day 5 count of Phase Three foods = 200 calories
Cumulative count of Phase Three foods = 700 calories

Day 6

BREAKFAST

Basic Egg White Omelette with mushrooms, spinach, onions, salsa, and ¼ cup (60 mL) shredded low-fat cheddar cheese
2 slices turkey bacon
Orange
Coffee with skim milk

LUNCH

Salad of mixed dark greens with turkey deli meat, cucumbers, tomatoes, peppers, and 1 tablespoon (15 mL) sunflower seeds
Green tea

DINNER

(If you love sushi, here is an example of how to fit it into your diet.)
Miso soup
Green salad
Salmon sashimi
6 spicy tuna rolls with ginger and light soy sauce—ask to hold mayo in rolls (**100 calories for the sushi rice**)
Orange

SNACK

Diet Fudgsicle™

Day 6 count of Phase Three foods = 100 calories
Cumulative count of Phase Three foods = 800 calories

Day 7

BREAKFAST
Basic Egg White Omelette with Asparagus, Feta, and Olives
Coffee with skim milk

LUNCH
The Best Homemade Chicken Soup
Veggies and fat-free dip

SNACK
Pretzels (2 oz/60 g) (**200 calories**), consumed with 1 12 oz (375 mL) glass of ice-cold water and flaxseed oil supplement

DINNER
Salad with tomatoes, cucumber, and sautéed wild mushrooms, with olive oil and vinegar dressing
BBQ ribs (4)
BBQ chicken
Steamed green beans with toasted almonds (in moderation)
Roasted red peppers

SNACK
Diet gelatin

Day 7 count of Phase Three foods = 200 calories
Cumulative count of Phase Three foods = 1000 calories!

PHASE FOUR

MAINTENANCE

You did it! You look great, and I bet you feel great too. So, how can you prevent the pounds from coming back? It's all about maintenance!

This lifelong maintenance phase is simple; it's virtually the same as Phase Three. The only difference is how you approach the foods introduced in Phase Two. These are the foods that are lower in water than those introduced in Phase One. During Phase Two you limited yourself to no more than three portions per day. But also recall that Phase Two foods are "hotty" and help to stabilize blood sugar and insulin levels; they are also great for the prevention of many medical conditions and ailments. So now that you have reached your goal weight, I encourage you to indulge in these healthy foods; you no longer have to limit yourself to three servings per day. Just use your weight as your guide. If it starts to climb a little, cut back. Soon enough, you will learn exactly what your body requires to stay healthy, thin, and gorgeous!

RESTAURANT RECIPES

Dr. Melissa Hershberg resides in Toronto. The following are a collection of delicious recipes contributed by some of her favorite restaurants and chefs in the city.

From the restaurant . . .

Didier

1496 Yonge Street, Toronto, Ontario
416-925-8588
www.restaurantdidier.com

EXECUTIVE CHEF: DIDIER LEROY

Cultivating his skills in fine and Michelin-starred restaurants in Toronto and Paris, Chef Didier Leroy emerged as the keeper of French elegance and simplicity. To dine at Didier is to be reacquainted with the classics of French elegance, prepared with impeccable technique and the finest Canadian, organic ingredients.

ঌ Waldorf Salad

This beautifully constructed rendition of the classic is sure to impress.
Makes 4 servings.

3	bunches mâche lettuce (small dark green-leafed French lettuce also known as corn salad)	3
1	medium celery root	1
	Juice of 1 lemon	
5½ oz	mayonnaise (can substitute fat-free or reduced-fat mayonnaise)	150 g
2 oz	Dijon mustard	50 g

3–4 dashes	salt and white pepper	3–4 dashes
2	Golden Delicious apples, cored, peeled, and cut into ¼- × 2-inch (0.5 × 5 cm) sticks	
1	package (2.6 oz/75 g) unsalted walnut pieces	1
	Walnut oil to taste	

Gently clean and dry lettuce and set aside.

Peel celery root, cut in half and grate into long strips. Place in a large bowl, squeeze in lemon juice and mix thoroughly. Add mayonnaise, mustard, salt and pepper. This is called Celeriac Remoulade.

In the center of the salad plate, fan mâche lettuce in a circle, stems in. Delicately place a large spoonful of remoulade in the middle and press down to flatten slightly. Arrange apple sticks on top, sprinkle with walnuts and drizzle with walnut oil.

Red Snapper en Papillote

Bursting with flavor and aroma; quick and simple to execute
Makes 4 servings.

4	fresh red snapper fillets, boned, skin on about 4 oz/125 g each	4
	Olive oil	
1	medium green zucchini sliced into ¼-inch (0.5 cm) discs	1
3	vine-ripened tomatoes, thinly sliced	3
8	medium button mushrooms, thinly sliced	8
1	bunch fresh basil	1
	Juice of 1 lemon	
	Sea salt	
	Freshly ground black pepper	

Preheat oven to 450°F (230°C).

Spread out four 8- × 8-inch squares of aluminum foil on working area, shiny side down. Drizzle olive oil in a small circle in the center of each square. Center and layer vegetables in a line, beginning with zucchini; follow with tomatoes, mushrooms, and basil. Lay snapper fillets atop, skin side up, and add a pinch of salt and pepper. Gently bring edges of foil in to form a small satchel. Do not close completely.

Bake in preheated oven or on medium-high barbecue grill for 8–10 minutes.

Present in foil, allowing guests to open foil bags themselves and drizzle fresh lemon juice and olive oil over the cooked fish.

From the restaurant . . .

Centro Restaurant & Lounge

2472 Yonge Street, Toronto, Ontario
416-483-2211
www.centro.ca

EXECUTIVE CHEF: BRUCE WOODS

Centro Restaurant & Lounge offers a liberating New American menu with impeccable five-star service (ask about their wine lockers). Chef Woods crowns his expertise with a diverse and approachable cuisine of superb meats and seafood, while offering a new-metropolitan mix of sushi, dim sum, tapas, and other small dishes in the lower-level lounge.

✆ Pan-Roasted Scallops with Charred Chilean Carica and Tropical Fruit Salsa
Makes 4 servings.

SALSA

1	whole Chilean carica* in syrup	1
¼	dragon fruit, peeled and chopped into ¾-inch (2 cm) squares × 4	¼
¼	avocado, peeled and chopped into ¾-inch (2 cm) square × 4	¼
¼	papaya, peeled and chopped into ¾-inch (2 cm) square × 4	¼

¼	red onion, peeled and chopped into ¾-inch (2 cm) square × 4	¼
¼	Thai chili, seeded and chopped fine	¼
2 tbsp	freshly squeezed lime juice	30 mL
2 tbsp	rice wine vinegar	30 mL
2 tbsp	syrup from the Chilean carica	30 mL
1 tsp	fresh coriander, roughly chopped	5 mL
2 tbsp	green onions, roughly chopped	30 mL
	Salt to taste	
	Freshly ground black pepper to taste	

SCALLOPS

8	large sea scallops	8
1 tbsp	canola oil	15 mL
	Salt to taste	
	White pepper to taste	

* The Chilean carica is a rare and unique boutique fruit that grows in the semi-desert areas of northern Chile. The flavor is like a combination of pineapple, mango, and peach.

SALSA

Drain the carica and reserve the syrup. Char the carica over a grill or in a smoking-hot pan lightly coated with canola oil. Let the carica cool, then roughly chop it. Combine with the dragon fruit, avocado, papaya, red onion, chili, lime juice, vinegar, reserved syrup, coriander, green onions, salt, and pepper and set aside at room temperature.

SCALLOPS

Preheat oven to 400°F (200°C).

Coat the scallops with canola oil and season with salt and pepper. Bring a thick-bottomed frying pan to smoking over medium-high heat (the pan must be hot to roast the scallops or the water will come out of the scallops into the pan, causing the scallops to boil and not caramelize). Cook the scallops on one side for approximately 30 seconds, undisturbed, to caramelize. Turn and cook for 30 seconds on the other side, then place them in the preheated oven for 3–5 minutes.

Remove the scallops from the pan, pat them dry on a clean towel and place them on a plate, 2 per person. Spoon some salsa on top of each scallop and serve.

From the restaurant . . .

MEATing

2411 Yonge Street, Toronto, Ontario
416-487-8609
www.meating.com

EXECUTIVE CHEF: SEAN SIMMONS

MEATing—A stylish modern-day interpretation of the traditional steak-house. MEATing's selection of meats change daily and features tame (farmed), game (wild), and organic (grain- and grass-fed). The menu also offers guests the choice of non-meat mains including vegetarian and seafood dishes.

∝ Veal T-Bone with European Steakhouse Seasoning and Pan-Fried Greens

Makes 1 serving.

1	Veal T-bone (14 to 16 oz/400 to 450 g)	1
1 tbsp	extra virgin olive oil	15 mL
	Sea salt	
	Cracked pepper	
1 tbsp	herbes de Provence *	15 mL
1 oz	asparagus, chopped into 1-inch (2.5 cm) pieces	30 g
1 oz	broccoli, chopped into 1-inch (2.5 cm) florets	30 g
1 oz	sugar snap peas	30 g
1 oz	snow peas	30 g

½ oz	olive oil	15 g
½ tbsp	cracked pepper	7 mL
½ tbsp	sea salt	7 mL

* Herbes de Provence is a spice mix commonly used in France to season chicken, veggies, or chicken. It can be bought already prepared or created at home by combining the following ingredients:

3 tbsp	dried marjoram	45 mL
3 tbsp	dried thyme	45 mL
3 tbsp	dried savory	45 mL
1 tsp	dried basil	5 mL
1 tsp	dried rosemary	5 mL
½ tsp	dried sage	2 mL
½ tsp	fennel seeds	2 mL

Can be stored in a tightly lidded jar for up to 4 months.

Veal T-bone
Preheat grill or broiler to high.

Brush veal T-bone with extra-virgin olive oil. Sprinkle herb seasoning on both sides of the veal. Place veal on high heat or under hot broiler. Cook for approximately 3 minutes a side for medium rare.

Let stand for 5 minutes.

Pan-Fried Greens
Heat olive oil in a sautépan over medium heat. Add asparagus and broccoli. Cook until tender (approximately 2 minutes). Add sugar snap peas, snow peas, pepper, and salt. Cook for 1 minute.

Place on a plate with T-bone and serve.

From the restaurant...

Mistura

265 Davenport Road, Toronto, Ontario
416-515-0009
www.mistura.ca

EXECUTIVE CHEF: MASSIMO CAPRA

Mistura restaurant offers contemporary Italian cuisine that reflects of a simplified yet refined approach to taste. The menu changes seasonally to ensure the freshest of ingredients and the best possible flavor.

✍ Winter Vegetable "Lasagna"
Can be served with Light Potato Cream for extra flavor.
Makes 4–6 servings.

LASAGNA

8	Savoy cabbage leaves, spine removed and discarded	8
1	Waxed turnip, washed, peeled, and sliced ⅛ inch (0.25 cm) thick	1
2	White onions sliced thin and lightly sautéed in oil	2
4	Garlic cloves, sliced thin and lightly sautéed in oil	4
1	Butternut squash, washed, peeled, and sliced ⅛ inch (0.25 cm) thick	1
1	Celery root (celeriac), washed, peeled, and sliced ⅛ inch (0.25 cm) thick	1
6	Green zucchini, washed, peeled, and sliced ⅛ inch (0.25 cm) thick (use skins only)	6

3	medium-size carrots, washed, peeled, and sliced ⅛ inch (0.25 cm) thick	3
1	Bunch Fresh thyme	1
4 tbsp	Extra virgin olive oil	60 mL
	Salt and freshly ground black pepper to taste	

Preheat oven to 400°F (200°C).

This lasagna is prepared by layering each vegetable on top of the other. Start with the cabbage leaves, add the turnip, then sprinkle with the onion and the garlic. Season each layer with salt, pepper, and thyme. Add the squash, the celeriac, more onion and garlic, the zucchini, the carrot, and top with more cabbage leaves. You may repeat the process once more for a taller lasagna. Bake in preheated oven for about 45 minutes and let stand for about 10 minutes.

LIGHT POTATO CREAM

2	large Yukon gold potatoes, diced into ¼-inch cubes	2
	Salt and freshly ground black pepper to taste	
	freshly grated nutmeg	
1 tbsp	butter	15 mL

LIGHT POTATO CREAM
Wash, peel, and finely dice the potatoes. In a saucepan, add water to about 1 inch (2.5 cm) over the potato. Season with salt, pepper, nutmeg to taste and butter. Simmer gently until completely cooked. With a handheld blender, purée until creamy, adjust seasoning and spoon on a plate to cover the bottom. Cut the lasagna into squares, put them in the middle of the plate and serve.

From the restaurant . . .

Lettuce Eatery

100 Wellington Street West (at York),
Toronto, Ontario
53 Bloor Street East, Toronto, Ontario
140 Spadina Avenue, Toronto, Ontario
130 King Street West, Toronto, Ontario
www.lettuceeatery.com

Lettuce Eatery is a hip and healthy quick-service food choice. It offers a large variety of ingredients and toppings to create delicious health-conscious meals that give customers the best "bang for the buck." The eateries are clean and modern, and the main focus is on serving made-to-order salads at an efficient and fast rate. Lettuce Eatery is based on a simple idea: prepare salads with the same quality ingredients, cooking techniques, and creativity found at the finest restaurants and serve them quickly, in a lively setting.

❩ Salad h2o

Makes 1 serving.

A bed of mesclun and iceberg lettuce, topped with chunks of blue cheese, grilled onions, Granny Smith apple slices, and smoked turkey—delicious with Honey Dijon Dressing (you may use your favorite brand or try the recipe below).

SALAD

2½ oz	mesclun mix	75 g
5 oz	iceberg lettuce	150 g
2½ oz	smoked turkey	75 g
1 oz	blue cheese	30 g
2¼ oz	Granny Smith apples	60 g
1¾ oz	grilled onion	50 g

Honey Dijon Dressing

1½ cups	low-fat or fat-free mayonnaise	375 mL
¼ cup	honey	60 mL
2 tbsp	minced onion	30 mL
2 tbsp	freshly squeezed lemon juice	30 mL
1 tsp	minced fresh parsley	5 mL
1 tsp	Dijon mustard	5 mL

Process all ingredients in a blender or food processor until smooth, stopping to scrape down sides. Cover and chill for at least 8 hours.

Serve over Salad h2o. Enjoy every bite.

From the restaurant . . .

Cfood

2419 Yonge Street, Toronto, Ontario
416-544-1661
www.cfood.com

EXECUTIVE CHEF: CHRIS MURIE

Cfood offers a modern, innovative, and delicious seafood dining experience. Committed to freshness and style, Cfood features a daily variety of simply prepared, fresh whole fish, filets, and other seafood.

▬ Pan-Seared Digby Scallops with Organic Niçoise Salad

Makes 2 servings.

4	Digby scallops	4
1	large pinch fragrant mint	1
1	small pinch fresh picked dill	1
1	bunch fresh chives, cut into small batons	1
1	small bunch baby frisée, cleaned and picked (use endive if not available)	1
2	organic eggs (hen or quail)	2
2 cups	light canola oil	250 mL
	Rinds of 2 lemons	
1	small pinch fresh lavender	1
¼ tsp	ground turmeric	1 mL

3	small organic potatoes (fingerling or baby new)	3
1	handful organic green beans	1
	Juice of 2 lemons	
½ tsp	Dijon mustard	2 mL
1 cup	baby heirloom tomatoes (cherry or grape)	250 mL
2	fine anchovies in brine (not oil)	2
	Coarse sea salt	
	Cracked pepper	

Cover the scallops and let them reach room temperature. Soak the mint, dill, chives and baby frisée in cold water in the fridge. Bring a small saucepot with salted water to a boil. Place eggs in boiling water (for quail eggs it should take about 3 minutes; for hen eggs 7 to 8 minutes). Immediately cool the eggs by running them under cold water when they are done. Once they have cooled, they can easily be peeled and should be stored in the fridge until needed.

In a small saucepan, combine canola oil, lemon rinds, lavender and turmeric. Place them on low heat and allow to simmer for 15 minutes. Remove from heat and let cool. Bring small saucepot to a boil with salted water; gently place potatoes into the water and reduce to a low simmer for 30 minutes, or until a fork will pass into them with ease. Strain and let the potatoes cool to room temperature.

Once again, bring the saucepot to a boil with salted water and blanch the handful of green beans for 3 minutes; then quickly refresh in ice-cold water to stop them from cooking further.

Remove mint, dill, chives, and frisée from water and let herbs drain on a paper towel. Strain the lemon rinds and lavender out of the canola oil, then combine your scented oil with lemon juice and Dijon into a smooth lemon-lavender dressing. Arrange the potatoes, tomatoes, green beans, anchovies and eggs on a plate. Season them with salt and pepper.

Bring cast-iron or nonstick frying pan to a high, smoking heat with a touch of light canola oil. While pan is heating up, season the scallops with salt and pepper. When pan is ready, drop the scallops on the hottest spots and allow them to sear for 90 seconds. Flip the scallops over, reduce the heat and let them sear on the other side for 2 to 3 minutes, depending on the size of scallops. Remove the scallops from the pan and allow them to rest for 2 to 3 minutes. Then place them on the arranged organic veggies. Top them with a liberal amount of herb blend and finish them with lemon-lavender dressing to taste.

From the restaurant . . .

The Boiler House

55 Mill Street, The Distillery District,
Toronto, Ontario
416-203-2121
www.boilerhouse.ca

EXECUTIVE CHEF: JASON ROSSO

The Boiler House restaurant offers a succulent chophouse-style menu with a breathtaking industrial chic setting.

✍ Pan-Seared Halibut on Chickpea and Sweet Corn Blanquette with Cumin-Scented Yogurt

Makes 4 servings.

HALIBUT

4	halibut fillet, (4 oz/125 g each), skin on	4
	Salt and pepper to taste	
1 tbsp	grapeseed oil	15 mL

BLANQUETTE

1 tbsp	grapeseed oil	15 mL
2 tbsp	garlic purée	30 mL
1	shallot, diced	1
1	yellow bell pepper, diced	1
1	red bell pepper, diced	1

1	bulb fennel, diced	1
1	English cucumber, diced	1
2	ears fresh corn, boiled, kernels removed	2
1 can	(19 oz/540 mL) chickpeas	1
1	red onion, diced	1
2 tbsp	chopped tarragon	30 mL
Splash	white wine	Splash

CUMIN-SCENTED YOGURT

1 cup	low-fat yogurt	250 mL
2 tbsp	cumin seeds, toasted	30 mL
2 tbsp	white balsamic vinegar	30 mL

HALIBUT

Preheat oven to 375°F (190°C).

Season the halibut generously with salt and black pepper; pan sear on high heat in a touch of grapeseed oil. Place in preheated oven for approximately 9 minutes.

BLANQUETTE

In a frying pan, on medium heat, add a touch of grapeseed oil and allow to warm. Add the garlic puree and diced shallot and sweat for 5 minutes. Add the yellow bell pepper, red bell pepper, fennel, cucumber, red onion, chickpeas, and corn; sauté for about 10 minutes. Add the chopped tarragon and a splash of white wine, cook dry and set aside. To finish, add 1 tbsp (30 mL) of the yogurt and season to taste.

CUMIN-SCENTED YOGURT

In a stainless steel bowl, add the yogurt; add the toasted cumin seeds and white balsamic vinegar. Mix very well and season to taste.

From the restaurant...

Toula Ristorante & Bar

One Harbour Square, 38th floor,
Westin Harbour Castle, Toronto, Ontario
416-777-2002
www.toularestaurant.com

EXECUTIVE CHEF: PINO PADULA

Declared by the Italian government as "the official ambassador of Italian cuisine in Canada," Toula offers classic northeastern Italian cuisine and a spectacular panoramic view of the Toronto skyline.

OCTOPUS SALAD

Makes 4 servings.

1 lb	octopus	450 g
1	bay leaf	1
1	celery stalk	1
½ cup	red wine vinegar, divided	125 mL
2	lemons	2
1	Cork from bottle of wine	1
1	Yukon gold potato	1
1 tbsp	extra-virgin olive oil	15 mL
	Salt to taste	
	Pepper to taste	

Place octopus in a pot with the bay leaf and celery and cover with water. Add a pinch of salt, 6 tbsp (90 mL) of the red wine vinegar (an espresso cup's worth, according to Pino), 1 lemon, halved, and the wine cork (this absorbs the acidity) and boil for 2½ hours. After it has completed boiling and has changed to a reddish color, remove the skin from the octopus (it should come off easily). Cube the octopus and the celery and set aside. Slice the potato into thin rounds and place it in boiling water for 2 minutes.

In a flat pan, lightly sauté the octopus, celery, and potato rounds in the remaining olive oil for 1–2 minutes with the remaining 2 tbsp (30 mL) red wine vinegar. Add salt, pepper, and lemon juice to taste.

⟋ Pear in Chocolate

Makes 4 servings.

4	Anjou pears	4
4 cups	dry red wine	1 L
2 tsp	sugar (can substitute Splenda)	10 mL
1	cinnamon stick	1
2 cups	chocolate sauce	500 mL

Remove the skin from the pears. Boil them in red wine with the sugar or Splenda and the cinnamon stick until the pears turn red. Drizzle lightly with chocolate sauce. Enjoy!

ACKNOWLEDGEMENTS

I would like to acknowledge the following people for their help, guidance and support.

To my agent, Rick Broadhead, thank you for your dedication, advice, hard work and steadfast belief in both my project and me personally from the very beginning. Your support and encouragement helped transform my vision into a reality and I am forever grateful.

Thank you to the entire team at Key Porter Books for your willingness to take a chance on a first time author. I am most grateful for your commitment to this project and for the many hours of hard work that were dedicated to it. A special mention and thank you to Jordan Fenn, Rob Howard, and Michael Mouland, whose advice, counsel, and intuitive grasp of the concepts underlying the manuscript were a great comfort and help throughout.

To all of the incredible chefs that contributed their wonderful recipes to the book, thank you for finding time in your unanimously frenzied schedules to participate in this project. Your recipes prove that healthy food can be as pleasing to our palettes as it is beneficial to our waistlines.

To doctors Bruce Topp and Susan Somerville, thank you for your unwavering support and encouragement and for allowing me to conduct the clinical research trial which offered proof of the diet's efficacy and acceptability amongst your patient population. I feel very lucky to have had the opportunity to work with you both.

Thank you to everyone who has reviewed and followed The Hershberg Diet. Your support, endorsements, testimonials, and stories of progress and success have meant the world to me.

I have been blessed with wonderful friends and family. To all of them, thank you from the bottom of my heart. You've shaped me, inspired me, nurtured me, motivated me, and put up with me—I love you all.

And to Tyler, my husband, partner, and best friend, this project would not have become what it is today without your help, advice, patience, love, and support. I am a better, stronger and smarter person because of you. Thank you for believing in me.

TRADEMARK INFORMATION

Specific products and name brands mentioned throughout this book are registered trademarks. The mention of trademarked products does not imply that the trademark holders endorse the Hershberg Diet.

All-Bran is a registered trademark of The Kellogg Company.

Bacardi White is a registered trademark of Bacardi and Company Limited.

Becel is a registered trademark of Unilever Canada Inc.

Bran Buds is a registered trademark of The Kellogg Company.

Coors Light is a registered trademark of Coors Brewing Company.

Creamsicles is a registered trademark of Good Humor-Breyers Ice Cream Company.

Crystal Light soft drink is a registered trademark of Kraft Foods Holdings, Inc.

Danone is a registered trademark of Groupe Danone.

Fibre 1 is a registered tradmark of General Mills Inc.

Fudgsicle is a registered tradmark of Good Humor-Breyers® Ice Cream Company.

Goldseal Tuna is a registered trademark of Canfisco.

I Can't Believe It's Not Butter is a registered trademark of Unilever United States, Inc.

Jell-O is a registered trademark of Kraft Foods Holdings, Inc., used under license.

McDonald's is a registered trademark of McDonald's Corporation.

Newman's Own is a registered trademark owned by No Limit, LLC.

PC Blue Menu Fibre First is a registered trademark of Loblaws, Inc.

Perrier is a registered trademark of Nestle waters North America.

Piller's is a registered trademark of Piller Sausages and Delicatessens Ltd.

Renee's is a registered trademark of Renee's Gourmet Foods Inc.

Silhouette is a registered trademark of Groupe Danone.

Splenda is a registered trademark of McNeil Nutritionals, a Division of McNeil-PPC, Inc.

Sugar Twin is a registered trademark of Alberto-Culver USA, Inc.